the Plant Clinic

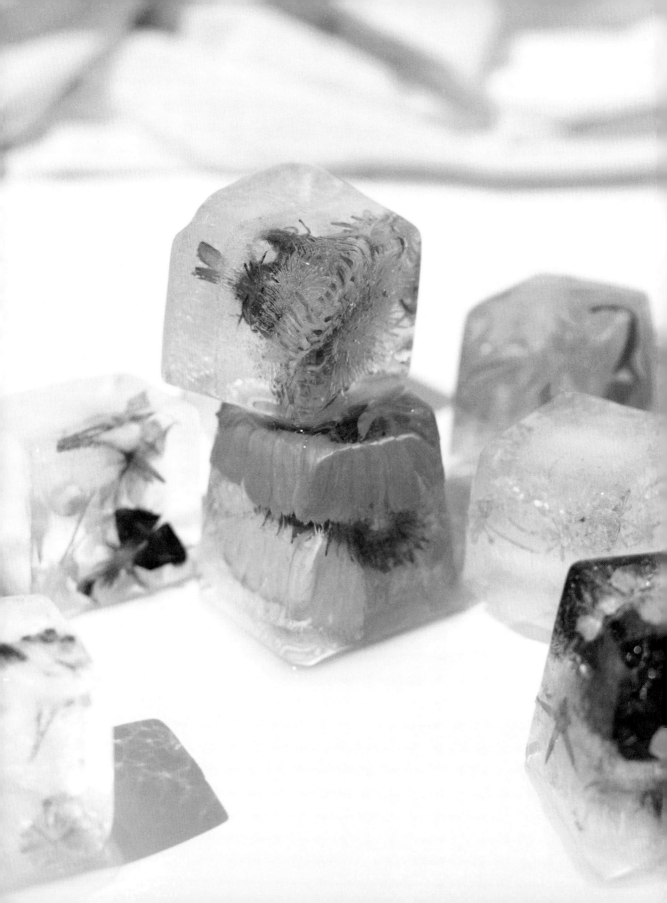

the Plant Clinic

Healing with plant medicine

ERIN LOVELL VERINDER

B Herb Med, Adv Dip Nut Med, Dip Energy Healing

Contents

Welcome to the Plant Clinic

Put simply, this is a love letter to living *vibrantly.*

Healing is no joke. It can be uncomfortable, messy and all-consuming, and it is certainly a nonlinear undertaking. The journey of healing is much like the metaphor of peeling an onion: healing lies within every layer, and as we peel each one back, we get closer to the heart. In uncovering the layers, we begin to change our perceptions and expressions of ill health. We awaken to see the patterns, the stories, the feelings held within ourselves.

As a clinical practitioner I witness all sorts of presentations, revelations, breakdowns and breakthroughs. Throughout any given week in clinic, there will always be a myriad of lovely clients sitting in front of me sharing their health stories, ranging from longstanding chronic conditions to acute complaints. I have learnt that my own health challenges and experiences have shaped me as a practitioner, and my ability to understand, guide and hold the space for others moving through their health challenges stems directly from my own experiences.

Years ago, I personally went through a terrifying chapter of burnout. I had been moving fast in many aspects of my life; emotionally I was frayed, physically I was weary. Changes needed to be made in my life. I felt the nudge of a physical symptom, yet I did not fully listen in. I have learnt the hard way that we often do this; as a coping mechanism, we ignore the messages of our bodies. Perhaps we cannot quite look at it or we aren't quite ready to hear it. We look away, wipe our hands of it, dust ourselves off and keep going. For me, this was a grave misstep.

My physical symptoms hit me like a bus. Literal waves of panic shook my body, yet my mind was still. Waves of anxiety washed through me. I was feeling out of my body, sped up and shaky. Cortisol rushes consumed me, and I really could not do much to keep them at bay. I went down allopathic treatment paths, with no answers and no solutions. I had no choice but to listen to my body, to make changes and to allow myself the space to heal.

Although the six Pillars to Thrive (p. 16) are age-old essentials, this is when I truly grasped the importance of these practices. In my own darkest moments, I dived headfirst into these practices to heal my body. I drank the water it was thirsty for. I balanced my blood sugar with nourishing food, eating with determined consistency to anchor my body. I connected to nature and let her fill me up everyday, swinging in my hammock under the trees and sitting in my garden. I moved my body ever so gently when I was able. I listened to my internal self-talk, adjusting each self-limiting thought with nothing but love and gentleness. And I rested. I rested so much; I cleared my calendar. It was not easy, but I knew I needed to. Healing demands a level of surrender, and surrender takes a whole new shape when you really face the true meaning of the word.

I leant heavily on plant medicine during this time, following my own plant protocols morning, day and night. Adaptogenic-rich herbals such as ashwagandha and rehmannia reshaped my internal stress response. Nervine-rich herbals such as passionflower, oat straw and skullcap helped to ground my nervous system. They were potent calmers of the cortisol rushes. They brought the light of hope with swift improvements and feelings of resilience returning. I got better very quickly. Within three months. This may seem like a long time, but when you are at rock bottom, a return to full vitality within three months is its own kind of radical.

While this experience truly brought me to my knees, it also offered me incredible insights and cracked open my life in a really wonderful way. I set a new pace, I now honour rest and know my limits lovingly, I lead with my heart and have learnt to not overextend myself. The whole breaking down to break through concept is quite literally the epitome of my (albeit messy) dance with burnout. Working with the plants allowed me to get to the very root of the issue. There was no shortcut or quick fix. I was worn so thin that I had to build from the ground up. This was deep healing.

In the Clinic

Unsurprisingly, I work with many burnt-out people. It is a natural side effect of our times, a modern epidemic of sorts. We have strayed far from the rhythms of nature, from a time when the simple rising of the sun and the setting of the moon were our compass. Instead, we wake to alarms and live our lives with various forms of technology dictating our daily movements and schedules. How can we all keep up?!

It's an incredible thing to watch clients return from the brink of brutal burnout with the assistance of restorative herbs and the Pillars to Thrive (p. 16). Often, one particular symptom, like poor energy, for example, improves with gentle interventions (such as herbs and rest), meaning fewer energy dips in the day; then sleep deepens, and gradually vitality is regained. This is the process of healing; one element affects another, and the pieces of your inner puzzle unite.

One client had been dealing with chronic bloating for a long time. She had tried every diet, had seen all sorts of medical specialists and undertaken invasive investigations with no results or improvements. After years, she turned to the plants. We discovered that her chronic digestive bloating was more a reflection of her internal emotional landscapes. Her response to stress was an inability to digest, a classic irritable bowel syndrome–like symptom. Once we had set up a herbal treatment plan – such as the Bloating Protocol on page 148 – to lean on, incorporating digestive herbs such as chamomile, lemon balm and fennel to calm her belly and her stress response, we had an incredible breakthrough. When her awareness shifted to working with plants to support her process, she transformed her bloating woes.

My own plant path has been an example of science and spirit finding their way back to each other. I am a Bachelor-level herbalist. My training was heavily clinical and science-based – involving the study of botany, anatomy and physiology, pharmacology, symptomatology, pathology and biochemistry of the body – alongside the sweet song of herbalism. However, when I embarked on the path of natural medicine as an eager teenager, my first learnt system of healing was energetic healing, with its esoteric view of health. Since

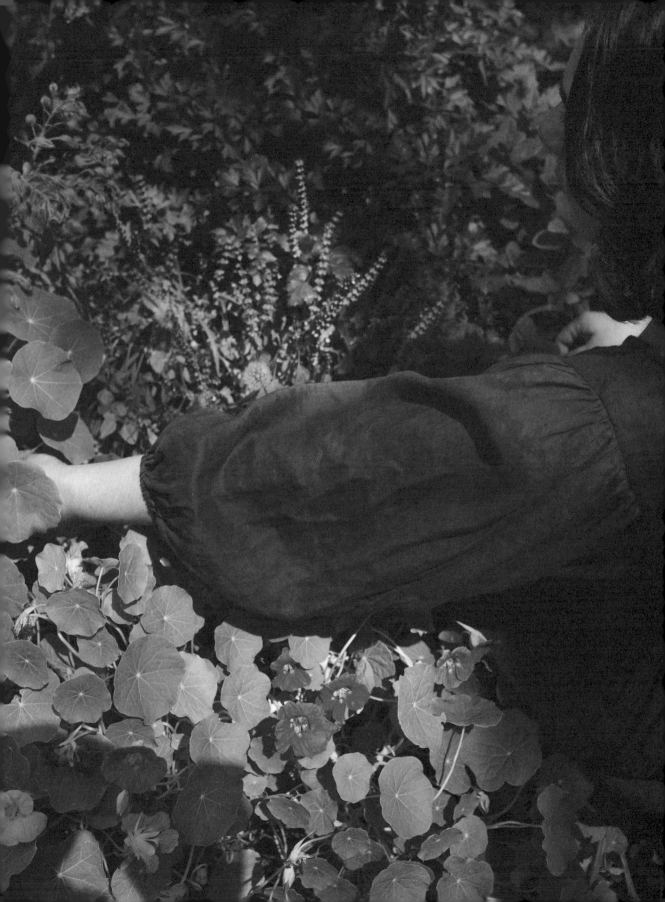

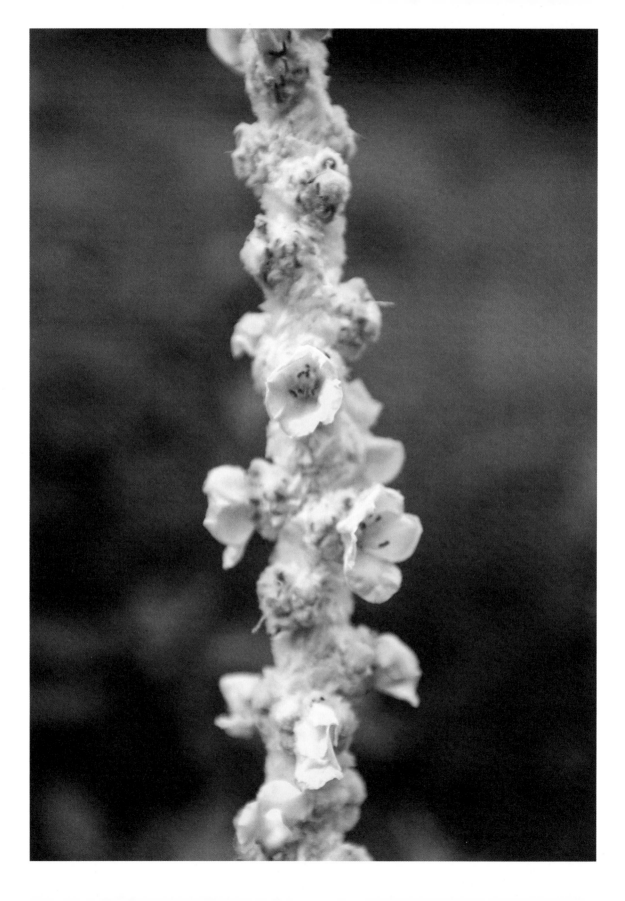

then, I have also dedicated years to my nutritional medicine studies, learning about the therapeutic benefits of food and the power in edible nourishment. I have merged my years of study and training with my years of clinical experiences, witnessing countless breakthroughs in my clients' ill health, working with them in restoring true health. What I am most certain of, is that you deserve to hold all of the tools that are needed to decode the messages being sent by your body and being.

Choosing the plant path takes us deep into the riches of traditional folk medicine and ancestral herbal therapeutics. We return to the old ways, marrying time-honoured approaches with contemporary practices and forging new ways to work with plants to heal our bodies and beings. The roots of herbalism run deep, and it is about time we found our way back to working with the plants to heal.

On finding your path as a plant *whisperer*

What I really want to illuminate about herbalism is that there are many dimensions to working with medicinal plants. In all honesty every herbalist will approach this slightly or even dramatically differently.

Ultimately this should be celebrated. The essence of herbalism is all about the individual's connection to the plants. I encourage you to approach plant medicine just as we herbalists do. Make it your own. Build your own connections and resonance with the plants.

The Power of the Plants

Plant medicine can work on so many different levels, and my aim is to educate and empower people to work with natural herbal interventions to positively impact their health on all levels. Plant medicine is a portal to reigniting whole health, throughout the body, mind and spirit. And, just as importantly, it offers a way back to nature, connecting your body and your being with the wisdom of the earth.

In essence, *The Plant Clinic* is a road map to wellbeing in the form of daily plant protocols and plant-based medicinal recipes, detailing a holistic approach to befriending your body with botanical healing. The protocols offer you structured daily guidance to support your return to true health. The corresponding herbal remedies elevate your healing routine to build and maintain health. You will find more than 150 plant-based remedy recipes in this book, many of them inspired by foundational naturopathic practices, grassroots herbalism and age-old folk wisdoms – applied alongside modern healing methodologies.

The way we can heal in relationship with plant medicine is wonderfully multifaceted, just as you are. When you experience the healing effects that plants impart, you begin to understand the magic that people and plants make together. There is an intelligence laced throughout the fabric of plant medicine, one that we cannot always quantify. One that offers adaptation – as we evolve, the plants evolve with us. The common thread is that plant medicine offers a refuge like no other. Operating in cahoots – nature's intelligence intersecting with our own innate wisdoms – the plants and the people make an incomparable duo. We humans are constantly shape-shifting and upgrading our way of living, and plant medicine is right there beside us in this unfolding. We, the modern folk, are ready to return home. To self, to nature, to enriched wellbeing.

Plant medicine has always been with us. The plants have long been present for the people. They are here to help us. Never limit a plant's ability to adapt to your needs; never limit your own ability to heal. This book is a reminder that the plants have got your back.

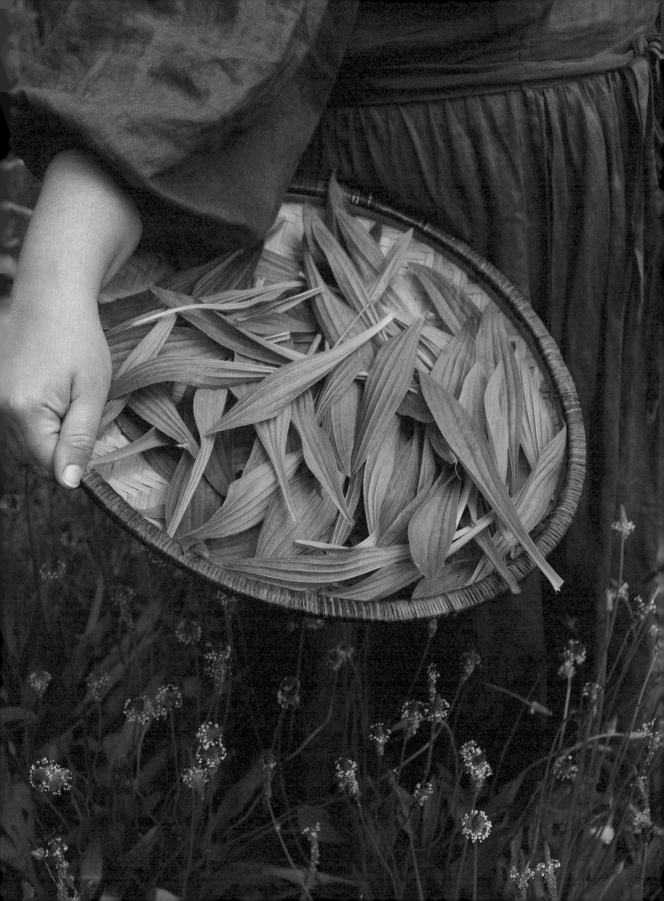

ON UNFOLDING

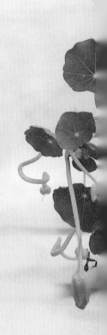

Often healing is not pretty. Sitting with discomfort is not easy. Sometimes you have to *break down to break through.*

Let's demystify the expectation of always being and feeling the same. Health is a representation of your evolution; it is *ever-changing.*

You are in motion. You are healing.

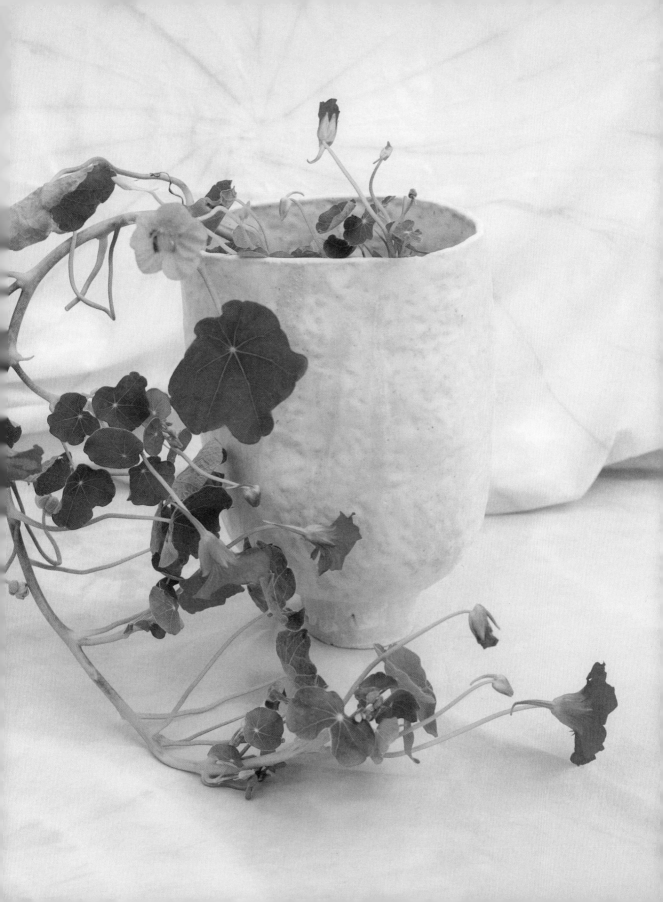

The Pillars to *Thrive*

The restorative power of the plants syncs with a deeper state of received healing when the body is hydrated, fed, grounded and in flow.

Being well means something different to each and every one of us. The idea of wellness is conceptual and, because of the endlessly varied standards we all hold, wellbeing is subjective and immeasurable. However, there are a few fundamental considerations that demand our commitment and attention in order for us to really up-level, support our own healing processes and embrace being well.

To potentise our relationship with any plant medicine and its application – to supercharge the process – we need to integrate the Pillars to Thrive: hydrate, good food, rest, body movement, self-talk and connecting with nature. These six pillars activate the physical, mental, emotional and spiritual bodies. In truth, they are non-negotiable building blocks for everyday vibrant health and wellbeing. You are about to meet the Pillars to Thrive. Lean on in – honestly, they are game changers.

1

Hydrate

Pure water hydrates our cells and enhances every function in our bodies. When you are hydrated, you feel clearer, more energised and more alive. The golden rule for hydration is 1 litre (4 cups) of water per 25 kilograms (55 pounds) of body weight. So, if you are 75 kilograms (165 pounds), you would aim to drink 3 litres (12 cups) of water daily. Ensure your water is filtered, and purified of heavy metals and contaminants, and opt for spring water where possible. Add a dash of pink sea salt to each litre of water – a simple way to enhance electrolyte replenishment.

The best way to remind yourself to stay hydrated is to get hold of a 1-litre glass bottle, keep it nearby and commit to refilling as needed!

2

Good Food

Nutrition is at the heart of our healing. What we choose to put into our bodies at every meal has a great impact on our overall ability to thrive. The particular way we approach food is inherent within each of us and was formed from our very first meals as little ones. Our relationships with food can be complex and layered. To further complicate this, everybody (and every body) needs a different, individual synergy of nutrition – there's no single diet that suits everyone! Some of you soar on a vegan diet, while others find animal proteins essential to feeling well. Either way, eating as mindfully as possible will benefit your overall health and healing process.

A balanced wholefoods diet with plenty of quality proteins, good fats, fibrous whole grains and a rainbow of fruit and veggies is the way to go. Choose local, and eat seasonal, organic and pesticide-free all the way where possible! Do your best not to get stuck on a fad; listen to your body and go with what feels good.

3

Rest

We need to rest. Period! Healing demands that we go within ourselves, to process, to integrate. Our bodies cannot consistently perform without reprieve. Rest is the safe harbour of peace we can offer ourselves when we are feeling weary. Vitality is found when our cup of energy is full to overflowing with nourishment; allowing ourselves restorative sleep and down time is essential if we are to recharge.

There are simple ways to do this, but begin by giving yourself permission to rest. You are no less wonderful or valuable for admitting to yourself that you need rest in order to balance out being a constant machine of doing (a by-product of the modern dilemma that confronts us all). Rest is a radical act of self-care.

Practise good sleep hygiene. Start simple: rest with the moon, rise with the sun. Consider your eating patterns and eat dinner early, at least 2 hours before bedtime; a full belly that is busily digesting makes it very difficult to sleep well. Power down all screens at least 1–2 hours before bedtime and remove all electronics from the bedroom to create a tech-free oasis! Suffuse yourself in a cosy, non-stimulating environment (low, warm lights, serene sounds and smells), particularly in the bedroom – keep it cool, quiet and dark. Lean into the mellowness of the evening with a book, a bath, journalling, meditation or good conversation. All of this will encourage the production of melatonin, our sleepy hormone, essential for a good night's rest.

4

Body Movement

Let's reframe exercise, okay? I think that exercise culture has, unfortunately, left many of us scarred. However, the truth is that moving your body daily is a quintessential part of wellbeing. Sitting is basically the new smoking, and countless studies show how a sedentary life leads to increased health risks and disease states. We need to move – to encourage energy to flow in and out of us, to activate muscles, to strengthen our cores, to lift our moods. Getting sweaty can actually be very fun. You don't have to run, you could dance; you don't have to join a gym, you could walk out in nature.

Check in with your energy on a daily basis and allow your choice of body movement to meet that level. It is an intuitive process, giving you room to make choices about how you want to move. If you are menstruating and don't feel super 'charged', go easy. If you are in an active state of healing, go extra gently. Remember, there are no rules, just a commitment to move daily in some way.

5

Self-Talk

How you speak to yourself impacts your ability to thrive and ultimately heal. Our thoughts impact our health: mind–body medicine is very real! Taking this into consideration, how can we 'show up' in our lives by using positivity and loving self-talk? A great place to start is to connect with the language we are using within, especially when we are in the process of actively healing our bodies. What are you telling yourself? Are you telling yourself you've got this, that you are healing? Or are you frustrated by your healing process and internalising your sharp tongue?

Reminding yourself that you are doing your best is so important when you are not feeling optimal and fantastic. Be gentle on yourself, praise yourself, perhaps weave in a daily affirmation. There is no need to impede your process of recovery with gnarly self-talk. Returning to gratitude (see p. 292) is a great way to reframe challenging situations.

6

Connect with Nature

Calibrating your body to the beat of nature is an essential part of inner and outer vibrancy. Adopting practices in alignment with nature is a sure-fire way to enhance your healing.

Connecting with nature harmonises our biological rhythms, encouraging balance and restoration. But we the modern folk are operating within a nature deficit, and the impacts of this are being felt on so many levels in relation to our health. Sun-ray phobia, for example, has paved the way for vitamin D deficiency, leading to many dire health consequences. Where possible, allow time and space for gentle sunshine-therapy sessions; this is an instant mood booster for most people, encouraging our body, with its innate intelligence, to synthesise those sun rays within itself. For an almost immediate, positive impact on stress, kick your shoes off and get onto the grass, onto the earth. This is an instantly grounding and rejuvenating practice for the senses.

Be sure to connect with nature daily in one way or another, be it a walk outside, time in the garden, a sun-kissed lunch break in the park or an evening gaze at the stars. Set a daily intention to be in nature. Even in the city there is nature all around us. All you need to do is look up to the vast canvas of the floating clouds and sky, and there she is – nature.

Food Is Medicine

We can choose healthfulness every time we make a meal. Here is a golden guide to get you inspired and connected to the power of food as medicine.

Diversify your internal ecosystem! Eating a wholesome diet will help you meet your required daily intake of proteins, beneficial fats and complex carbohydrates. There isn't a part of you that won't benefit from a broad, balanced diet. Bring on these stellar elements to really optimise your nutritional intake:

— **Protein:** Including protein-rich sources (animal- or plant-based – think grass-fed meats, legumes, tempeh, nuts, wild-caught fish, seeds, eggs, etc.) in every meal and snack helps to stabilise blood sugar, which in turn will help regulate your energy levels, vitality and hormonal balance. Protein is essential for our bodies to heal!

— **Fibre:** Found in fruits, veggies, legumes, nuts, seeds and whole grains, fibre is essential for a healthy gut. Increase your fibre intake to aid digestion and promote the clearance of internal waste products, which will help your gut and skin alike. Chia seeds, flax seeds and whole oats are awesome fibre-dense options to weave in for an extra dietary boost.

— **Fats:** Say yes to (good) fat! Unsaturated and monounsaturated fats are nutritionally rich and loaded with essential fatty acids that will not only boost your overall health and vitality but can particularly benefit your skin health, hormonal health and emotional wellbeing.

Welcome in olive oil, avocado, nuts, seeds, eggs, ghee and wild-caught oily fish such as sardines and mackerel. Many of these foods (especially fish, chia seeds, flax seeds and walnuts) are rich in omega-3, a fatty acid that's great for your skin, mood and gut.

— **Prebiotics:** These are fibres and sugars that stimulate good bacteria in your gut. Everyday prebiotics include garlic, onions, leeks, apples, asparagus, Jerusalem artichokes, legumes, lentils, honey and under-ripe bananas. Certain herbs are also a wonderful source of prebiotics such as dandelion root, marshmallow root, chicory root, slippery elm bark, elecampane root and burdock root.

— **Probiotics:** Bring on the fermented foods – all the pickles, all the sauerkraut, all the kefir! Probiotics are living microorganisms that promote the health and growth of gut flora to aid digestive health. If you are new to these foods, introduce them slowly and gently, so you can monitor how well you tolerate them. Miso, natto, cultured yoghurt, kimchi and wild-fermented vegetables are other great sources of probiotics.

— **Culinary spices, herbs and therapeutic foods:** Weave these into your cooking and supercharge your daily diet by incorporating healing foods, such as onions and garlic, in your meals – with antibacterial properties galore, they are incredibly powerful in assisting immune defence. Bring on culinary spice herbals such as dill, caraway, fennel, ginger, thyme, rosemary, oregano and turmeric to elevate the flavour of your dishes and add extra medicinal elements to your meals. Many of these herbals also have a remarkable impact on the gut and are antioxidant-rich stars!

— **Cooked vs raw:** When you are feeling burnt out and under the weather, steer away from raw, airy foods, such as salads. Although raw foods are super nutritious, to refuel your tank and rebuild internal vitality, lean into more grounding, warming, nourishing foods, such as broths, soups, stews, curries and congee.

— **Greens:** Eating a rainbow of vegetables is always encouraged, but getting your daily greens is key for your body to sparkle! Alongside your medley of everyday greens (spinach, chard, etc.), consider adding in liver-loving foods such as cruciferous veggies (broccoli, kale, Brussels sprouts), romaine lettuce, rocket (arugula), beets and bitter greens.

Remember to avoid skipping meals and pay attention to your pattern of energy spikes and slumps – including noting any dreaded 'hangry' episodes, when your blood sugar dips. Do your best to course-correct with regular wholesome meals and hearty snacks if needed.

IRRITANTS

A number of pro-inflammatory foods are part of many people's everyday diet. Consider eliminating or reducing as many as you can, where possible, to aid your health and wellbeing. These foods are notorious gut-irritants and hormone disrupters, and are typically troublesome for the skin, mood and overall vitality. Known pro-inflammatory foods and beverages include:

— **Processed foods:** Bad news all around. Often filled with refined sugars and complex saturated fats, processed foods are (ironically) not easy to process and can overload the body, causing inflammation.

— **Fatty fried foods:** Many of the saturated oils in which these foods are cooked are problematic for the skin, and the nature of fried foods aggravates the digestive system, particularly the liver and gall bladder.

— **Gluten and dairy:** Even if you're not necessarily intolerant to these common allergens, they can be hard to digest. Dairy in particular can exacerbate skin conditions, especially acne, and can be mucus-forming; avoid it if you're under the weather or battling a break-out. Many people are sensitive to gluten – if you suspect you are, give yourself the gift of a gluten-free reprieve for a few weeks and see how your body responds!

— **Caffeine, refined sugar and alcohol:** The rapid highs and lows of these stimulants and depressants leave the body's systems reeling. Both caffeine and alcohol can irritate the gut, as well as promoting dehydration and being common skin irritants. Alcohol also depresses the central nervous system and can wreak havoc on the evenness of our mental and emotional states. Taking a hiatus from caffeinated drinks, alcohol, chocolate and refined sugars is strongly recommended, even outside of focused detoxes, especially if you're feeling burnt out and they feel too speedy for your body. This will help you regain your balance, allow your true energy to repair and avoid pushing your body into an unnatural 'high'.

How to Use This Book

A GUIDE TO DECODING SYMPTOMS

Messages from the body could be in the form of

A physical symptom	**An emotion**	**A mind state**
e.g. a sore throat, aching legs, heavy cramps, a headache	e.g. feeling sad, anxious, angry, frustrated	e.g. feeling ungrounded, uncertain, negative, heavy

All of these can present in an interconnected manner and may be hard to separate. That is absolutely okay – you are a complex, multilayered being. The main thing is to tune into your body to work out which symptom you most need support for, then follow the appropriate daily protocol. You may start off following a protocol in the Hair and Skin section. After a while, once you begin to peel back the layers, you may find yourself moving on to Emotions, Mind, Spirit. *The Plant Clinic* will guide you through your entire health journey.

No two people will experience the exact same presentation of a symptom. The protocols, recipes and healthful suggestions that you will find in this book are a solid place to begin, but please allow this body of work to be malleable for your own needs and healing process. You can chop and change recipes, mix and match to suit the areas where you are needing the most support, and bring in the medicinal plants required by your body's unique healing journey.

Although there are herbal dosing guidelines on page 40, you must let your symptoms be the guiding light as to how the plant medicines are working for you, because the way you choose to apply a plant medicine – and the effects that you feel – will be entirely unique, your own symphony of healing in companionship with the plants. Plant medicines have an astonishing ability to adapt to all bodies in one way or another. When you try a plant medicine, ask yourself: how does it feel for me? The answers that may follow will lead you deeper into healing.

DAILY PROTOCOLS

Protocols are a day-by-day guide to return you to health. These tried-and-true protocols will assist you in finding your way back to your centre. I have refined these protocols over many years and present them here in their simplest, most effective and accessible form. Find yourself within the protocol descriptions and identify how and where your body is speaking to you, then experiment. There is plenty of room within the gentle prescriptive landscape ahead for you to make these protocols your own. When following the protocols, please keep in mind that there are no fixed timeframes when healing. Acute symptoms, such as a sore throat, generally resolve within a few days. If symptoms do not shift swiftly, it is wise to seek professional advice. More chronic symptoms, such as burnout, can take their time – be persistent and consistent, the results will come!

BASE RECIPES

Base recipes form the foundation of herbal medicine-making. They provide a blueprint for endless variations. For example, the steps to making an overnight infusion or an oxymel will always be the same, it's just the choice of herbal ingredients in the remedy recipe that determines whether it's a **Lush Locks Infusion** (p. 256) or a **Nutritive Overnight Infusion** (p. 194).

Many of these base recipes are rooted in easy-to-follow folk methods. For the sake of all you alchemists and kitchen herbalists out there, I have intentionally simplified these base recipes to make them totally accessible for you!

Please note that there are a few self-contained remedy recipes that do not require the use of a base recipe.

REMEDY RECIPES

The remedy recipes are a treasure trove of condition- or concern-specific medicinal recipes. For each remedy recipe, you will need to add the herbal ingredients to the appropriate base recipe foundational ingredients. Simply follow the type and quantity of plant material (and other ingredients) given in the herbal ingredients list of each remedy recipe.

Give these plant-rich recipes a go, to support and lift, restore and recalibrate.

A NOTE ON GENDERED TERMINOLOGY

There is often heavy usage of traditional gendered terms in herbalism and healing – 'for the woman', or 'for the man'. My take is that herbs are not gender-specific or binary. They work beautifully and efficiently for all bodies in different spheres and scenarios. It is time to up-level our concepts of plant medicine for all bodies. Aside from the two sections that concentrate specifically on female-focused care – Mums and Bubs and Hormonal Health – every recipe and health suggestion in this book extends to each and every one of you.

MEDICINE MAKING

FRESH OR DRIED INGREDIENTS

You will notice that the remedy recipes mostly call for dried plant ingredients over fresh. There are a couple of reasons for this.

— **Accessibility:** Dried plants are easy to access. They are available in health food stores, dispensaries and online.

— **Longevity:** Dried plants are easy to keep on hand in a home apothecary. They can be stored simply and safely – ideally, sealed in an airtight glass jar and away from direct sunlight in a cool, dry cupboard. Dried plant material is also far less problematic than fresh when you are making plant medicines. Although beautiful to work with, fresh plants can present challenges such as mould formation and spoilage (particularly common in herbal oils), and often demand a little more trial and error during the preparation process.

If you do choose to use fresh plants, double the recommended amount given in the recipe for dried herbs. There are some plants that really are best to work with fresh, and I have noted these where relevant in the remedy recipe.

SOURCING PLANT MATERIAL

Non-organically grown plants will have been sprayed with many potentially harmful chemicals. When the plant material is steeped in a small amount of water – as in a tea, for example – the chemical residue becomes condensed. It is highly advisable to source organically grown plant material from reputable growers and stores. Where possible, opt for locally grown plants; working with plants in tune with the land you stand on brings an extra level of synergy. Growing your own plant medicines can also be incredibly rewarding, representing an opportunity to get to know the plants intimately. For easy access, there are many reputable online retailers offering an incredibly extensive array of dried herbs, and health food stores also generally stock them in abundance.

CONSUMING CONSCIOUSLY

We must activate our consciousness when we consume anything, including plants.

We live in community with plants, and we are sincerely responsible for our impact on their wellbeing and longevity. As herbalists, we need to lead by example, so that this great green Earth of ours lives on vibrantly and the passage of herbal wisdom continues to be passed on from one generation to another.

Whether you are a novice or an expert, it is truly your duty to be mindful of where the plants actually come from and how they came to be with you. A great place to begin is by asking these few key questions and actively seeking answers:

— Where did this plant grow, and was it grown sustainably?

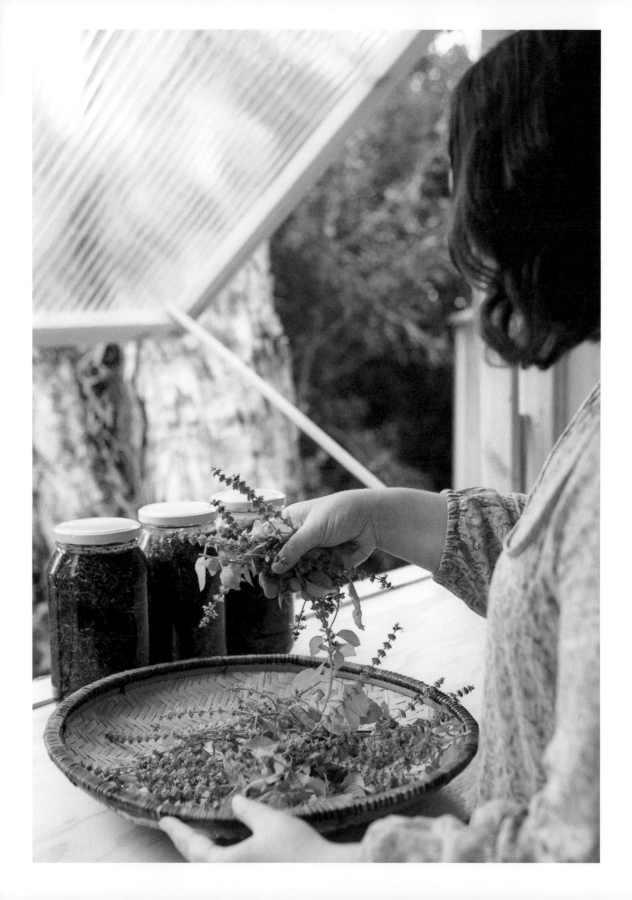

— Is this a rare/potentially at-risk or endangered plant? If so, can I work with another more sustainable plant medicine instead?
— How far did this plant material travel to be with me?
— Can I utilise more plants grown locally within my region/country?

We may not always get the full answers we are seeking, but it is so important to inquire, in order to support conservation efforts and eco-conscious practices.

Or, even better, grow your own!

DRYING PLANT MEDICINES

There are multiple ways to dry fresh medicinal plants. Air-drying is a premium way to dry plants and maintain their medicinal magic. One method involves simply tying a bunch of plants at the base and hanging them up to air-dry in a well-aerated, warm space out of direct sunlight. You can also air-dry your fresh plants on baking trays lined with cheesecloth, turning the plant material daily. Be sure to keep your trays in a warm spot away from direct sunlight. The plant material usually takes 4–5 days to dry fully.

Alternatively, if you have a dehydrator, you can set it to the lowest 'living food' temperature (35°C–45°C/95°F–115°F); the precise temperature will depend on the humidity present in your environment. For example, you may need to increase the temperature if there is high humidity in the air. Spread the plants out evenly on the dehydrator trays and set to dry for

between 4 and 12 hours – the drying time really depends on the type of plant material. Ensure your plants are completely dry, with no moisture present, before you go ahead and seal and store them in glass jars.

STERILISING JARS AND BOTTLES

Many of the recipes in this book call for you to mix and/or store your plant-powered potions in sterilised glass jars or bottles. This ensures that any harmful bacteria, yeasts or fungi are banished from the vessels before you fill them with your finished remedies. I use two simple methods, which are listed below. And a little extra tip: try to sterilise your glass vessels as close as possible to bottling time.

— **Stovetop:** Fill a large saucepan with cold water and submerge the jars and lids in the pot. Bring to a full boil, then reduce the heat to medium and keep at a consistent boil for 10 minutes. Remove the sterilised containers and lids, and allow them to air-dry.

— **Dishwasher:** Use the hottest cycle to sterilise your vessels. When the cycle is complete, remove the jars and lids, and allow them to air-dry completely.

STORING PLANT MEDICINES

The shelf life of dried herbs varies widely, so employ your senses to check their freshness. How they smell, taste and appear is the best way to gauge their viability and medicinal life force. The best way to store your herbals is in airtight, sealed glass jars that should be kept well away from direct light – in a cool, dark cupboard is ideal. We herbalists generally prefer to bottle our dried herbs, tinctures and salves in amber-toned glass to keep them unspoilt and extra fresh.

A NOTE ON ESSENTIAL OILS

You will notice that I rarely add essential oils to my recipes. This is deliberate. It takes an incredible amount of plant material to make a tiny bottle of essential oil. And so, with that knowledge, and in the spirit of consuming consciously, I suggest using herbal oil infusions rather than essential oils. Of course, essential oils pack a mighty punch, as they are constituted of incredibly condensed plant material. But often a simple oil infusion will work just as well, reducing the need to use extreme amounts of plant material in the creation of remedy recipes.

Equipment list

Here are a few essential and helpful items to assist your medicine-making endeavours. Recipes will highlight the specific equipment needed.

— Baking paper
— Baking tray or brownie pan
  (20 x 20 centimetres/8 x 8 inches)
— Candy or chocolate moulds (silicon)
— Candy thermometer
— Capsule maker
— Capsules (size 00; vegetable-based or
  gelatin-based)
— Cheesecloth or muslin
— Coffee or spice grinder
— Cotton cloth (soft)
— Double boiler
— Fine-mesh sieve, large
— Fine-mesh sieve, tea leaf strainer
— Food processor
— Glass bottles, dropper bottles and jars of
  all sizes with lids (amber bottles and jars
  are extra wonderful for reducing sunlight
  exposure and extending longevity)
— Handheld kitchen mixer
— Heat pack or hot-water bottle
— Heatproof glass bowls
— Heatproof mason jar (1 litre/4 cups/
  34 fluid ounces)
— Immersion blender
— Milk frother
— Mortar and pestle
— Mugs and cups that you love to drink from
— Neti pot
— Saucepans, small to large
— Scissors
— Spoons (wooden and metal) for mixing and
  measuring
— Teapot

Base Recipes

These base recipes form the foundations for your herbal medicine-making. They have been intentionally simplified to make them as accessible as possible, but as you become more skilled you will find that your confidence in experimenting will expand. I wholeheartedly encourage you to play, create and make these recipes your own.

Candies

MAKES 20 CANDIES

Candies taste really good, there is no doubt about that! These portable plant-rich gems are also truly medicinal for sore throats, coughs and congestion. Pop them in a little tin and take them as needed to usher in honey-laden relief. They do pack a sweet punch, so be mindful of your herbal candy intake.

First, make ¼ cup of strong medicinal tea infusion with the herbal ingredients, brewing the tea for at least 20 minutes before straining through a fine-mesh sieve. Add the infused tea base and 1 cup of honey to a heavy-bottomed saucepan and simmer over medium to high heat. It's best to use a candy thermometer here, as the mix needs to get to around 150°C (300°F). This will take around 25–30 minutes. If you do not have a thermometer, you can test if the candy is ready by dropping a little of the mixture into ice cold water. If the mixture is ready, it will harden instantly! Do be very careful, though, as hot sugar burns can be very serious and very sore.

Once ready, pour your candy mixture into small silicon moulds (any mould will do, but the candies are much easier to remove from silicon) and allow to cool completely. Remove from the moulds and dust with your herbal powder of choice (such as the rose petal powder in the **Calm Candies** remedy recipe, p. 278). You can roll each candy in baking paper for freshness and portability, or store sealed in an airtight container for 2–4 weeks. If you live in a warmer climate, keep these in the fridge!

Capsules

MAKES 50 CAPSULES

Capsules are a quick route to downing your daily dose of herbs. Easy to swallow and portable, they also allow you to bypass the flavour of some undeniably ghastly-tasting herbs! It may seem a little intimidating to make these at home – but, really, it is simply about getting your herbal powder into a capsule. You can do this one capsule at a time, or if you want to make larger quantities of capsules, invest in a capsule maker! Vegetable- or gelatin-based capsules are perfect options, and size 00 is ideal, holding around 500–700 milligrams powdered herb per capsule.

Pop your prepared plant powder into a small, sterilised bowl, then decant into the bottom section of an open capsule. Fill the bottom section halfway to the brim, then secure the bottom and top sections of the capsule together. Seal capsules securely in a sterilised jar and store in a cool, dark, dry place away from direct sunlight and heat.

Decoctions

MAKES 3 CUPS

Decoctions are simply simmered, water-based medicinal teas made from hardier, woodier plant parts, such as roots, rhizomes, twigs, barks, berries and mushrooms. These require more time and enduring heat to coax out their medicinal constituents. Decoctions are best drunk within 48 hours and should be kept in the fridge to maintain freshness.

Add your herbal ingredients and 5 cups cold water to a saucepan. Bring to a rapid boil, cover and reduce to a simmer for 20–30 minutes. The water will reduce significantly in the boiling process, so feel free to top up with extra water if needed. Remove from the heat and allow to cool to drinking temperature before straining through a fine-mesh sieve to serve.

Electuaries

MAKES ¼ CUP

Essentially, an electuary is a medicinal paste made of ground plant powders mixed with honey. Honey is liquid gold, and once infused with herbs it becomes an alchemical nectar! Aromatic herbs work particularly well – think chamomile, rose petals and lavender. Be sure to use a good-quality, bee-friendly raw honey as your base, as it offers a wealth of beneficial enzymes. Electuraries store well and are an easy, ready-to-use remedy for the home apothecary – they can can be added to hot water to make instant sweet tea, drizzled over foods and eaten straight off the spoon.

In a sterilised bowl, pour ¼ cup raw honey over the powdered herbal ingredients. With a clean spoon, mix the honey and powders until well combined. Decant the herbal honey into a freshly sterilised jar. Seal the jar with an airtight lid and label, noting the ingredients, remedy recipe name and date made. Store in a cool, dark place, or in the fridge.

Glycetract Extracts

MAKES 1–2 CUPS
(Depending on the dried herbs used)

Glycetract extracts are alcohol-free tinctures, made with a food-grade vegetable-glycerin base. They are a great alternative method of extracting medicinal constituents, at the same time offering a sweetened base. Glycetracts are great for children and those sensitive to alcohol, and have a thick, sweet, syrupy nature that most people take to instantly! They can also taste quite delicious, making them a perfect remedy for an irritated throat or a cough. Many people prefer to use glycerin-based extracts over alcohol extracts, and a tincture recipe can generally be transformed into a glycetract extract with ease! Please note that there are many ways to make glycetracts to efficiently extract a plant's medicinal elements. For ease, we are keeping it real simple here!

Begin by making up your menstruum – the liquid solvent that acts as the tincture base to draw out the medicinal plant constituents. To make 2 cups of menstruum, mix 350 millilitres (12 fluid ounces) of food-grade vegetable glycerin with 150 millilitres (5 fluid ounces) of distilled water in a sterilised jar, seal it with a lid and shake thoroughly until well combined.

Finely chop the dried herbal ingredients or grind them in a spice grinder and place them in a separate sterilised glass jar. Pour the menstruum over the chopped dried herbs, filling the jar right to the top. Seal the jar with an airtight lid and allow to sit for 4–6 weeks, giving it a little shake and good energy every day or so. In cooler climates you will need to allow the full 6 weeks, but in warmer climates 4 weeks should be absolutely fine.

When the extract is ready, strain out the plant material by pouring the glycetract through a single layer of cheesecloth. You may need to strain twice if fine plant material is still present in the extract. Squeeze out every last drop of the menstruum from the cloth. Decant the glycetract into sterilised amber glass bottles. Seal and label, noting the ingredients, remedy recipe name and date made. The general shelf life of a correctly stored glycetract is around 1–2 years.

Herbal-Infused Oils

MAKES 1¹/₂–2 CUPS
(Depending on the dried herbs used)

Herbal oils offer a deep well of nourishment for the skin, forming a base for making balms, salves, creams, massage oils and body butters. They are a true gift to incorporate into your self-care practice – once you start making and working with these oils, you will never look at pre-made skincare products the same way! Herbal oils are generally best made with dried plant material. Fresh plants can often be the cause of mould or spoilage if moisture is present, and can be trickier to navigate if you are new to oil infusions.

First, coarsely chop your herbal ingredients into small pieces. Add the plant material to a sterilised glass jar and fully immerse it in 2 cups carrier oil (olive, almond, sunflower or apricot kernel oil are perfect due to their high omega-9 oleic acid content), leaving a 5–8 centimetre (2–3 inch) space at the top. Push down the plant material with a sterile knife to release any air pockets and to create a little more room in the jar for extra oil to be added. Completely covering the plant material with oil protects against oxidation and spoilage.

Seal with an airtight lid, label and store for 4–6 weeks. Visit often and give the jar a gentle shake, checking that the plant material remains covered by the oil. You will notice that the oil gently changes colour, taking on the elements of the infused plant. When the oil is ready, strain it through clean cheesecloth, muslin or a large fine-mesh sieve and decant the infused oil into a sterilised jar. Seal tightly and label, noting the ingredients, remedy recipe name and date made.

Lather these oils directly onto the skin to nurture and moisturise, or use them in skincare and topical herbal product recipes.

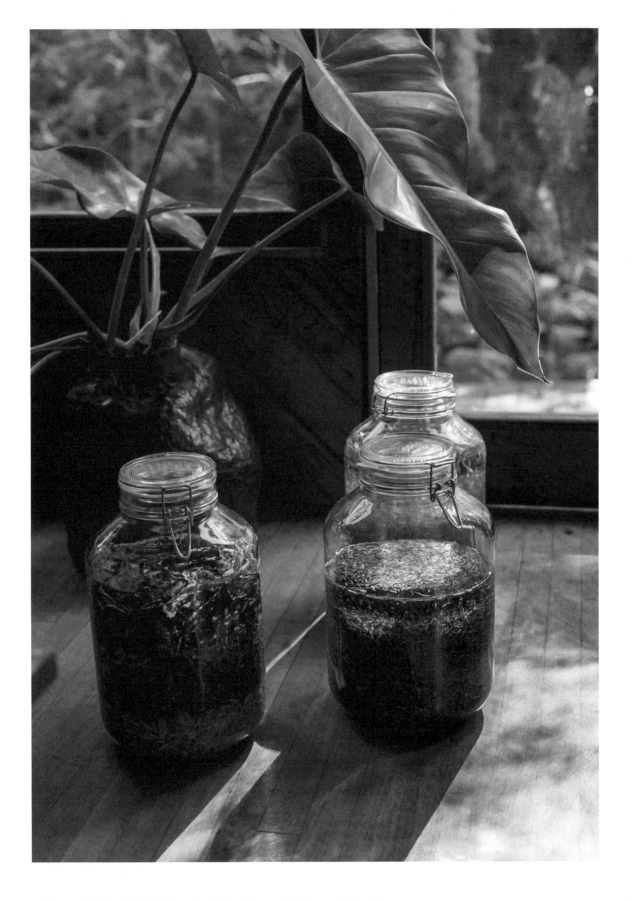

Herbal Powders

MAKES ½–1 CUP
(Depending on the dried herbs used)

Powders are a really great way to include more plants in your diet and are easily made using any dried herbs you have handy. If you are using whole herbs, you will need either a mortar and pestle or a spice grinder to grind them into a fine powder. Be mindful when you are grinding down your dried herbs that oxidation can occur when the plant material is exposed to the air, shortening the shelf life of your herbal powders. It is best to make smaller batches, which can be utilised as needed.

Place your dried herbal ingredients in spice grinder or mortar and pestle and grind to a fine powder. Decant into a sterilised jar with an airtight lid. Seal and label, noting the ingredients, remedy recipe name and date made.

Simply add the powders to your water bottle, smoothies or plant mylk tonics, make them into a capsule, or use them as a base for a salad dressing or add to cooked meals.

Medicinal Teas

MAKES A SMALL TO MEDIUM POT (ABOUT 3 CUPS)

Quite simply, medicinal teas are made by steeping and infusing your plant material in water to create a herbal brew. Softer plant parts, such as flowers, leaves, stems and buds, are particularly suitable for use in teas. Deepen the medicinal powers of the plants by allowing them to brew for longer. Medicinal teas are best drunk fresh, so keep them in the fridge and drink within 24 hours.

Place your herbal ingredients into your teapot. Add 3 cups boiling water and put the lid on the teapot. Steep for 10–20 minutes before straining through a fine-mesh sieve to serve.

Overnight Water Infusions

MAKES 4 CUPS

Deepen your experience of drinking the plants with a slow-brewed overnight water infusion. Essentially this is medicinal tea that is infused for an extended period of time to gently extract minerals, vitamins and beneficial plant constituents. Overnight infusions are best made with softer plant parts: flowers, leaves, stems and buds. I find the easiest way to bring this practice on board is to prep before bedtime, leave to infuse overnight and then enjoy it the next day.

Pop your herbal ingredients into a sterilised 1-litre (4-cup) heatproof mason jar. Pour in 1 litre of boiling water and seal the lid. Leave to cool and infuse for a minimum of 4 hours and a maximum of 10 hours, before straining through a fine-mesh sieve to serve. If you prefer a warm infusion, gently reheat in a saucepan on the stove to the desired temperature.

Oxymels

MAKES 2–3 CUPS
(Depending on the dried herbs used)

One of the most beloved and delicious forms of plant medicine. Super foolproof, with raw honey and apple cider vinegar as the base extraction ingredients, oxymels create a tasty 'tincture meets syrup'. Oxymels also make the very best spritzer when added to fizzy water! They are a great alternative for those seeking to avoid alcohol-based herbal tinctures.

Place your dried herbal ingredients in a sterilised glass jar. Pour 2 cups of raw, unpasteurised apple cider vinegar over the plant material, followed by 2 cups of raw honey. The liquid mixture should completely cover the plant material and fill the jar to the very top. Seal the jar with a plastic lid. If you are using a metal lid, place a piece of baking paper between the mixture and lid before sealing to avoid any corrosion. Allow your oxymel to infuse for 2–4 weeks.

When the oxymel is ready, simply strain it through a fine-mesh sieve, pressing the dried plant material with a spoon to liberate the liquid. Decant the oxymel into sterilised amber bottles. Seal and label, noting the ingredients, remedy recipe name and date made. Oxymels store well at room temperature, but if you live in a hot climate you can extend their longevity by keeping them in the fridge.

You can add oxymels to carbonated water, use them as a healthful cocktail/mocktail base, add them to smoothies or herbal teas or just drop them straight onto the tongue!

Plant Mylk Tonics

MAKES 1 CUP

This milky elixir is usually enjoyed warm, but is equally awesome drunk over ice. Plant mylk tonics are an outstanding way to include powdered herbs and medicinal mushrooms in your daily diet. Simply pair your herbs or mushrooms with a store-bought or homemade mylk, whether that be coconut, nut-based (such as almond or cashew) or seed-based (such as hemp or pumpkin).

A milk frother really comes in handy if you are regularly making tonics, helping to thoroughly marry the liquid and powders to minimise grittiness. However, you can achieve an equally delicious result by heating your tonic in a saucepan on the stove.

To make a warm mylk tonic, add the herbal ingredients and 1 cup plant mylk together in a milk frother and set to 'warm', or heat gently in a saucepan. If adding raw honey as a sweetener, ensure that your tonic is not boiling hot, as excess heat will degrade the honey's beneficial enzymes. Once warm, pour into your favourite mug, dust with a little cinnamon, sip slowly and savour the warmth.

To make a cold mylk tonic, add the herbal ingredients and 1 cup plant mylk together in a milk frother set to 'cool', or blitz in a blender. Then simply pour into a tall glass over ice, sprinkle with edible petals and enjoy.

Poultices

When you need a super-quick method of applying plant material to the skin, poultices are the way to go! Incredibly easy to master, a poultice can be made with dried, powdered or fresh herbs. The poultice can be directly applied to the skin to offer relief from bites, scrapes, rashes and much more.

First, make the paste or pulp. If you are using dried or powdered herbs, add a little hot water to make a paste. If using fresh plants, simply chop them into a pulp. The paste or pulp can then be directly applied to the area in need.

Note: An alternative method – which is helpful for strong heat-giving herbs such as ginger – involves sandwiching the paste or pulp between two pieces of clean, soft cotton cloth before the cloth is placed on the affected area. This method avoids any direct contact between the poultice and the skin. It is recommended in the **Ginger Poultice** *remedy recipe (p. 187).*

Salves

Salves are true saviours for the skin! They soothe irritations, dermal cuts, scrapes and bruises, combat skin dryness and offer a portable way to take your plants with you wherever you may go! Salves are semi-solid, softening once rubbed into skin, and are simply made from a herbal-infused oil and beeswax base (beeswax is undeniably nourishing and healing for the skin). Once you have your herbal oil ready, you can make salves with ease.

Make your Herbal-Infused Oil (p. 31) ahead of time. This forms the base for your salve.

Place ¼ cup beeswax pastilles (chopped wax is also fine) and 1 cup of your herbal-infused oil in a double boiler over medium heat. Alternatively, place them in a heatproof glass bowl over a saucepan filled with boiling water. Allow the beeswax to melt and combine with the herbal oil, stirring gently. This usually takes 2–4 minutes. Once the beeswax has melted, remove the saucepan or bowl from the heat source and swifty add any essential oils, if you're using them, to the liquid mix. Then quickly pour the salve into sterilised amber glass jars or tins. Allow the salve to cool completely and harden before covering the jar or tin with the lid and sealing. Label, noting the ingredients, remedy recipe name and date made. Store in a cool, dark, dry place to prolong the longevity of your salve. It will happily last 1–2 years! If you prefer a firmer, balm-like salve, simply increase the amount of beeswax.

Syrups

Simple Syrup
MAKES 2 CUPS

Slow-Brew Syrup
MAKES 4 CUPS

Syrups are the most delectable method of delivering plant medicines. Adults love them and kids love them – compliance is usually very high when a medicinal syrup is on offer! There are many ways to make a syrup, but I suggest using these two versions as you begin your medicine-making endeavours: one is a simple syrup and the other is a slow-brewed version. You will see in the remedy recipes that each syrup calls for a specific technique. If you are vegan, you can sub out the honey and use brown rice syrup instead.

To make a simple syrup, first make a strong medicinal tea using 2 cups water, infusing the tea for at least 20 minutes before straining through a fine-mesh sieve into a heatproof bowl. Add 1 cup raw honey to the bowl and mix gently with a wooden spoon until the honey melts through. As the infusion will be only mildly warm at this point, the beneficial enzymes in the raw honey will be unaffected by the heat. Pour the syrup into sterilised bottles, allowing it to cool completely before sealing. Label, noting the ingredients, remedy recipe name and date made, and store in the fridge for 1–2 months.

To make a slow-brew syrup, place 2 cups of water, ¼ cup of black strap molasses, 7 ½ cups sugar-free fruit juice (I recommend pomegranate juice or cherry juice concentrate) and all of the herbal ingredients outlined in your remedy recipe straight into a large saucepan. (Do not include the raw honey; it will be added later in the process.) Bring the mixture to a boil over medium heat, then reduce the heat to low. Allow to simmer, stirring occasionally, for 1 hour or until reduced by almost half, then remove from the heat. Allow the syrup to cool to a lukewarm temperature, strain out the herbal ingredients (and compost them, ideally!), then stir in 1 cup raw honey and ½ cup brandy (optional). If you like your syrup extra thick, you can always pump up the honey content!

Leave the syrup to cool completely and then decant into sterilised bottles. Seal securely and label, noting the ingredients, remedy recipe name and date made. Store in the fridge for up to 6 months. Although the brandy helps to extend the shelf life, it can be omitted. Note that your syrup will only stay fresh for 1–2 months without the alcohol content.

Tinctures

MAKES 2 CUPS

Tinctures are an incredibly important part of any apothecary, enabling herbalists to deliver medicinals with ease – and to customise formulas for all sorts of health concerns. Tinctures are often made from one single herb with an alcohol base. With its ready availability, 80-plus proof vodka is a perfect menstruum; it also has a neutral taste and the ability to act as a broad solvent. Many of the remedy recipes in this book are blended multi-herb tinctures, with a number of herbs added to a single tincture preparation; this method simplifies the medicine-making process and yields a complete, customised plant-medicine formula. Tincture making can get super complex, but the pared-back folk method outlined below is incredibly easy to follow. Please note that the tincture remedy recipes call for dried herbs, which has dictated the suggested quantities. If you want to use fresh herbs, as a general rule double the amount specified in the remedy recipes.

Finely chop your herbal ingredients or grind them in a spice grinder and place them in a sterilised glass jar. Pour 2 cups of your chosen menstruum over the plant material, ensuring the herbs are completely covered and filling the jar right to the top. To avoid any mould formation, the plant material must remain completely covered with the menstruum. Seal the jar well with an airtight lid (if you are using a metal lid, place a piece of baking paper between the menstruum and lid before sealing to avoid any corrosion) and store for 4–8 weeks, visiting often to give it a good shake and good energy! Be sure to keep the herbs completely covered with the menstruum so that they macerate effectively. Note that some types of plant material will absorb alcohol, so you might need to top up with a little more menstruum.

When your tincture is ready, strain into a clean container through a slightly dampened double layer of cheesecloth. Be sure to squeeze out every last precious drop of menstruum! Decant the tincture into sterilised amber glass bottles. Seal and label, noting the ingredients, remedy recipe name and date made – if stored correctly, they will have an indefinite shelf life.

Vinegars

MAKES 2 CUPS

Herbal vinegars are simply herbs infused in a vinegar base. Vinegar is an awesome liberator of medicinal constituents, drawing out beneficial plant extracts with ease! Vinegars have long been used in herbalism, offering a handy way to work with all types of herbs, from fresh to dried. They are entirely flexible: they can be used for culinary endeavours or taken neat off the spoon. I recommend using raw apple cider vinegar as the foundational ingredient here – it has many healthful benefits for the gut and beyond, and yields a tasty vinegar time and time again.

Add your dried or fresh herbal ingredients to a sterilised glass jar. Pour 2 cups of vinegar over the plant material, filling the jar to the top and ensuring the herbs are completely covered. Seal the jar with a plastic lid. If you are using a metal lid, place a piece of baking paper between the mixture and lid before sealing to avoid any corrosion. Shake well and store for 2–6 weeks. When the vinegar is ready, strain through a fine-mesh sieve and decant the vinegar into sterilised glass bottles. Seal and label, noting the ingredients, remedy recipe name and date made. Herbal vinegars will have greater longevity if stored in the fridge.

Use your vinegar to snazz up a salad dressing, as a marinade or drizzled over roasted veggies. Or you can add it to bubbly water for a zingy spritzer or even just take a spoonful straight up.

Washes

MAKES 1 CUP

A wash is essentially a water-based medicinal tea used topically on the skin. It's perfect for instances when a quick intervention is needed, such as cleaning a cut or scrape, or for washing smaller areas of the body, like the face or the eye region.

Prepare your wash as you would a Medicinal Tea (p. 33). But we want the wash to be concentrated, so reduce the water used in the base recipe to 1 cup. Once brewed, allow it to cool to a comfortable temperature before pouring into a clean bowl. Dip a cotton pad into the wash and allow it to soak up the infused liquid. Press and wipe the pad onto the areas in need. Use a fresh cotton pad for every wash immersion – do not double dip. You can keep your wash fresh for up to 24 hours by storing it in the fridge.

Guidelines for Dosing Plant Medicines

Given that dosing is quintessentially geared to meet the needs of a specific individual, offering a blanket approach is challenging. Herbs are not drugs, so basing all dosages on weight, much as pharmaceuticals do, comes with limitations (with the exception of the formula shared on page 43 to help you navigate kids' dosing). It is important to take into consideration the potency of the herb, the individual's constitution, and the severity of the presentation and symptom. I am offering these general guidelines to point you in a solid direction as you begin working with the recipes that appear in the following section. But the most golden advice I can give you is to start with a lower dose and then tune in to how your body feels in response to the plant medicine preparation – from there, you can increase the dosage as needed. Often, if someone feels a plant remedy is not working, it is simply because the dose is 'off' and needs an adjustment.

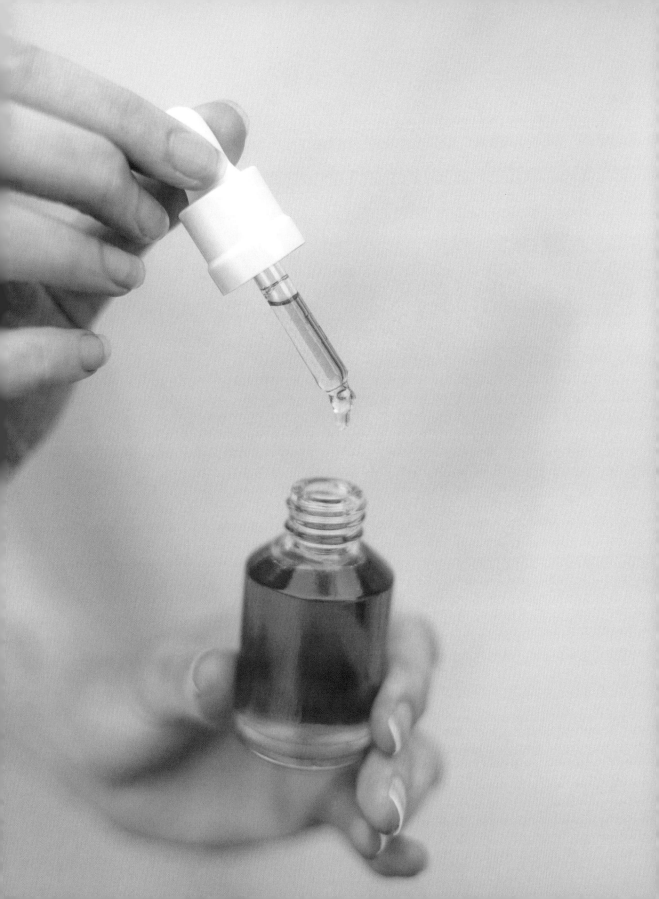

Constitutional considerations

For ease, I would love you to ask yourself
if you resonate or lean more towards
one or the other of the following folk.
Knowing this can be super helpful when
working with and dosing plant medicines.

Robust folk

— Are you unfazed by smells, tastes
  and stimuli?
— Do you struggle to notice any
  differences when taking herbs and
  supplements?
— Are you an extroverted, living-life-
  large person?

Sensitive folk

— Are you sensitive to smells, sounds,
  tastes and stimuli?
— Do you notice that you are
  very responsive to herbs and
  supplements?
— Are you a quiet, naturally
  introverted person?

If you identify with the robust folk, you may
need to dose your plant medicines a little
on the higher side. If you identify with the
sensitive folk, you may need to dose your
plant medicines a little more towards the
lower side.

ACUTE DOSING

When you are experiencing sudden-onset,
swiftly intensifying (acute) symptoms – as
with a cold, for example – it is important
to support these acute presentations
by dosing your plant medicines more
frequently until they abate.

CHRONIC DOSING

When health concerns and symptoms linger
without improvement, or worsen over time,
it is important to dose your plant medicines
consistently and to work with your remedies
for a longer period of time in order to clear
chronic concerns.

EVERYDAY DOSING

For a healthful approach to working with
plant medicines – when it is not so much
about an acute or chronic presentation but
more a quest for wellbeing support – follow
the everyday dosing suggestions. Consider
the herbs as healing tonics for your day.

DROP DOSING

This practice is based on small 'drop doses' of herbs, using a dropper – as compared with higher dosing, which is far more commonly suggested in modern herbalism literature. Drop dosing shines light on the immeasurable power within the plants, taking a far more esoteric stance on the unquantifiable, unseen forces that the medicinal plant holds within itself. I can share with you that drop dosing tiny amounts of medicinal remedies works profoundly well for many of my clients in practice. Plant magic strikes again!

More is not always better when it comes to plant medicine dosages. Where did that idea even come from, I wonder? The concept of less is more can be a powerful ethos to support you and yours when it comes to consuming plant medicines. The beauty of utilising low doses is that this approach is entirely sustainable; it will prolong your apothecary stores and can be employed for plants that are rare and/or at higher risk of extinction. Experiment, and find your dosing groove.

DOSING FOR CHILDREN

Dosing little ones with herbs – and doing so with confidence – can be exceptionally challenging. It is so important to tread cautiously and take an extra level of care!

This is why I follow Clark's rule – a reliable, long-employed formula – when calculating dosing for children (of all ages). Please remember that children do very well with gentle, low dosing; consider drop dosing for the young folk.

Clark's rule is based on weight, and is always calculated using imperial rather than metric measurements.

— Begin with the recommended adult dose, which is based on a 150-pound (68-kilogram) adult – generally a standard adult dose.
— Measure the child's weight in pounds.
— Divide the child's weight by 150 and multiply by the adult dose.

For example, if the child weighs 70 pounds, and the adult dose is 3 cups, the dosage would be 1.4 cups of the recommended adult dose (70/150 = 0.46 x 3 = 1.4 cups).

A NOTE ON HONEY FOR INFANTS

Honey, which is used in a variety of recipes, is not suitable for infants under the age of 12 months.

	Acute Adult Dosing	Chronic Adult Dosing	Everyday Adult Dosing
Body Butters	*Not commonly used in acute presentations	Apply one to three times daily	Apply once or twice daily
Candies	Up to 6 candies throughout the day	*Not commonly used in chronic presentations	*Most commonly used in acute presentations
Capsules	2–4 capsules three times daily	2–4 capsules once or twice daily	2 capsules once or twice daily
Electuaries	1 teaspoon three times daily	1 teaspoon twice daily	1 teaspoon daily
Glycetract Extracts	$\frac{1}{2}$–$\frac{3}{4}$ teaspoon four times daily	$\frac{1}{2}$–1 teaspoon three times daily	$\frac{1}{2}$–1 teaspoon two to three times daily
Herbal-Infused Oils	To keep the skin moist, lather areas in need up to three times daily	To keep the skin moist, lather areas in need up to three times daily	To keep the skin moist, lather areas in need up to three times daily
Herbal Powders	*Not commonly used in acute presentations	1 teaspoon three to four times daily	1 teaspoon twice daily
Medicinal Teas/ Decoctions	$\frac{1}{2}$–1 cup hourly until acute symptoms ease	3–4 cups daily for at least 12 weeks	1–4 cups daily
Overnight Water Infusions	*As for medicinal teas	* As for medicinal teas	* As for medicinal teas

	Acute Adult Dosing	Chronic Adult Dosing	Everyday Adult Dosing
Oxymels	1 teaspoon four times daily	1–2 teaspoons twice daily	1 teaspoon once daily
Poultices	Apply to areas in need two to three times daily	Apply to areas in need one to three times daily	*Most commonly used in acute or chronic presentations
Salves	Apply topically, hourly, to areas in need	Apply topically as needed, generally two to four times daily	*Generally used for acute or chronic presentations
Sprays	Spray on areas in need hourly until symptoms ease	*Most commonly used in acute presentations	*Most commonly used in acute presentations
Steams *excluding pelvic steams*	Two to three times daily	Once or twice daily	*Most commonly used in acute or chronic presentations
Syrups	1–2 teaspoons two to three times daily	1–2 teaspoons twice daily	2 teaspoons once daily
Tinctures	½–¾ teaspoon four times daily	½–1 teaspoon three times daily	½–1 teaspoon two to three times daily
Vinegars	1 teaspoon four times daily	2 teaspoons twice daily	1–2 teaspoons once daily
Washes/Rinses/Baths	One to three times daily	One to three times daily	*Most commonly used in acute or chronic presentations

Note: Plant mylk tonics are not included in the above table as they do not have a specific dosage and can be enjoyed freely.

Vitality

Vitality and energy are kin; when I speak of vitality, I am making an implied reference to the concept of energy and the animation of the spirit. To refer to 'vitality' in isolation from energy is to misunderstand the true essence of the word. Our inherent life force – our vital force – is held within and exudes outwards. In effect, each of us embodies an incandescent force-field; we as beings are energetic, and this vital force is responsible for our wellbeing in many ways. Understandably, it is challenging to gauge intangible concepts like radiance and health. Yet there are many ways in which vitality can be fed and upgraded – and when the mind, body and spirit are strong, we are full of vitality.

Being vital is most definitely a feeling. I often ask my clients to tune in to how they are feeling in their body and being when we have our session, offering them a scale ranging from 0 (absolutely flatlined, no energy present), to 5 (energy is there, but really only just functional, just getting by) and up to 10 (ecstatic, awesome energy). I wonder, where are you sitting on the scale? This potent exercise enables you to tap into the levels of energy/vitality within and activates your awareness of any low points in your day; for example, the common 3 pm slump, when we reach for a sweet treat or a pick-me-up to help us shake off the weariness.

There are many ways to combat low energy, and most of these remedies stem from a deeper practice of healthfulness. Surprisingly, it can be quite simple to increase vitality. Actioning and increasing conscious breath (oxygenating the body) and drinking pure water, eating wholesome foods, allowing yourself to rest, bringing on supportive body movement, keeping a positive attitude and immersing yourself in nature are all powerful allies. Medicinal plants will lend you potent assistance as your stepladder upwards and onwards to a wellspring of energy.

Seemingly complicated (and, admittedly, sometimes actually very complicated) health complaints such as insomnia, fatigue, lacklustre energy and low libido are all intertwined and are often dependent on vitality. Although the topic of libido frequently crosses over into hormonal imbalances, it has a LOT to do with innate vitality. When someone is stressed, exhausted – just a shell of their usual selves – the spark-dependent fervour of the libido is often flatlined. As we restore vitality and energy, the fire can return!

If you find yourself repeatedly returning to this section, it is time to lean in to the ancient intelligence of the Pillars to Thrive (p. 16). It is also your cue to turn to adaptogenic herbs and soothing concoctions to refill the cup of vitality and illuminate your life force, so that you can shine bright like a diamond.

Consider these elements essential to reviving vibrancy

— Balance your blood sugar (see p. 208). Be sure to include a protein source with each meal and snack; this can be animal- or plant-based to suit your dietary choices.

— Ground a burnt-out body with beneficial fats (see p. 20). Weave them into your daily meals and snacks.

— Remove all stimulants (see p. 21), especially if you are feeling tired or wired.

— Include lots of vibrant, seasonal fruits and veggies – in other words, eat the rainbow (see p. 21).

— Keep up hydration (see p. 17). Water makes your cells sing with gusto, and you will feel brighter when you are well hydrated.

— Rest! (see p. 18)

Burnout

Upon Rising	Morning and Afternoon	
DRINK a tall glass of room-temperature water mixed with a teaspoon of spirulina or chlorella and an optional squeeze of fresh lemon juice, if you like. These nutrient-dense algae add a flush of chlorophyll-rich energy that provides a balanced (not-too-buzzy) boost.	**DOSE UP** on the **Adrenal Rebuilder Tincture: Formulas 1 and 2** (p. 56), containing oats, ashwagandha, rhodiola, tulsi, passionflower and Siberian ginseng. Choose the formula that matches your symptom presentation.	
Enhancements	**CONSIDER** bringing in supplementation to assist burnout recovery. A great B complex, vitamin C and magnesium are majorly indicated here. Address any underlying nutrient deficiencies such as low iron or B12, get your bloods tested and work with your practitioner to create a guided supplement plan.	

Burnout masquerades under many monikers. It is often referred to as adrenal exhaustion or adrenal fatigue. Whether there is a functional issue with the adrenal glands or, more correctly, with the HPA axis (hypothalamic–pituitary–adrenal axis), burnout is a collection of symptoms that are deeply felt by many people. Fatigue can be experienced on several levels – physical, mental and emotional – and in the case of burnout, each of these states will generally be depleted and malfunctioning. Time to restore, dear ones. Bring this protocol on board as a daily practice.

Throughout the Day	Evening
SIP the gentle yet remarkably impactful **Nettle and Oat Straw Infusion** (p. 68), to support nourishment of deep fatigue, ground the nervous system and rebuild vitality.	**DRINK** a double-strength brew of **Chamomile Tea** (p. 161) after dinner, to usher in sweet sleep.

PRACTISE THE PILLARS

REST. I cannot stress this enough. Rest is the essential healer of burnout; claim it whenever possible. Eat really **GOOD FOOD**. It is critical to balance your blood sugar by eating every 2–3 hours. Aim for protein-dense snacks and meals, and eat the rainbow – fresh, nourishing food. You really cannot skip this step if you wish to heal burnout. Food is your medicine. Practise **SELF-TALK**. Connect with the inner conversations you may be having about allowing yourself rest and healing. **CONNECT WITH NATURE**. One of the most profound ways to heal burnout is to be with the plants, the ultimate source of life. They will remind you of the route to regeneration.

Insomnia / Poor Sleep

Throughout the Day	Evening
SIP the caffeine-free **Zen Day Tea** (p. 73), a peaceful blend of oat straw (to centre your nervous system) and adaptogenic tulsi (to regain equilibrium).	**POP** **The Dream Duster** (p. 58). Take these capsules with your dinner. The trio of passionflower, chamomile and skullcap will pave the way for a good night's sleep. *and/or* **DROP** a dose of the **Slumber Drops** (p. 69) before bed, to gently sedate your body if you are feeling restless or wired. This tranquil extract of kava root, reishi and rose petals will induce bliss in the astral realms.

Sleep is deeply interconnected with our vitality. If we do not sleep, we become shells of our usual selves. Whether it is fleeting or chronic insomnia, sleeplessness can be the most jarring and tormenting experience, a repetitive battle with the dark of night. There are many factors that impact a sound night's sleep, ranging from your stress levels, to your environment, to the foods you are eating. It is important to take stock of all of these elements in order to usher in sound sleep and ensure you are practising good sleep hygiene. Luckily for us all, there are many plants that can influence our ability to sleep well, offering the chance to form a healthier relationship with sleep. Bring on the herbal night caps!

Enhancements

PRACTISE THE PILLARS

REST: sleep hygiene, sleep hygiene and more sleep hygiene! Bring on **BODY MOVEMENT**. Exercise is a perfect way to expend energy and rewire the sleep cycle. Rise with the sun, sleep with the moon – **CONNECT WITH NATURE** and let her show you the way. **SELF-TALK** can get fairly charged when you are facing sleeplessness and mounting frustration around lack of sleep. Bring on a mindfulness practice, such as meditation, to quieten the mind and welcome in a softer dialogue.

CONSIDER

all of the elements that may impact poor sleep – see the guidelines for sleep hygiene (p. 18).

DAILY PROTOCOL

Longevity

Morning	Throughout the Day
POP the **Supreme Shrooms** capsules (p. 121), a blended medicinal-mushroom complex with superstar longevity abilities. *or* **DROP** a dose of the **Timelessness Tincture** (p. 73), to enhance the life force and longevity. This neuro-enhancing adaptogenic tonic combo embraces many of the most revered herbs, including the 'herb of immortality', gynostemma.	**DRINK** **Live Long and Prosper** (p. 63), to support vitalism. This antioxidant-laden iced herbal cocktail will transport you to a tropical moment with green tea, hibiscus, lemon peel, turmeric and goji berries. *or* **SIP** **Bright Eyes Tea** (p. 57), a tart brew that assists with vision and embraces the antioxidant-rich goodness of bilberries, while gently supporting the liver with calendula and cornflower. This tea blend is also quite literally eye candy ... so beautiful.

It is time to harness the ancient ways in which herbs have been utilised to support longevity. Not only do these medicinal plants aid your external health, more importantly they nourish the internal landscape of health. To enhance your natural radiance and life force, braid these antioxidant-rich herbal tonics and vital plants into your everyday. Be mindful that there is no magic pill to halt the ageing process. But there are many plant medicines and lifestyle interventions that can assist in supporting a strong mind, body and spirit – which will certainly increase your ability to live well and age well.

Enhancements

PRACTISE THE PILLARS

Bring all the Pillars to Thrive on board for a long, happy, healthy life!

EAT

an increased amount of vitality-enhancing herbs. Add turmeric, ginger and cinnamon aplenty to your cooking.

Low Libido

Morning	Afternoon and Evening
### DRINK the lively **Lush Loins Tonic** (p. 65), laced with the libido-enhancing medicinal mushroom cordyceps and triumphant maca root. A super-delicious libation to kick-start the day. ### POP **The Awakener Caps** (p. 57), an adrenal-system boost in capsule form. Made with the root-rich trio of ashwagandha, licorice and Siberian ginseng, this uplifting blend can reignite the spark within for weary and depleted folk.	### SPOON **The Lovers' Oxymel** (p. 64) onto the tongue for a tangy, honey-drenched, spirited jolt of aphrodisiacal plant medicine.

This protocol sits in the vitality section, as low libido is a natural by-product of stress, exhaustion and lack of innate vibrancy and vitality. Yes, absolutely, hormonal imbalances can be a causative factor, but more commonly in this modern day there is an interconnection between a loss of inner sparkle and a low libido. When experiencing lacklustre energy, stress or a sense of mental or emotional compression, generally the last thing anyone wants to do is give themselves over to another, passionately! Addressing the underlying factors – like deep levels of burnout or hormonal imbalances – is also key, but working with medicinal libido-awakeners, aphrodisiacs and adaptogens is a wonderful way to rekindle fervour and sensuality.

Enhancements

PRACTISE THE PILLARS

REST well. Eat GOOD FOOD. HYDRATE aplenty. Get in touch with your luscious temple (your body!) with BODY MOVEMENT. Fill your cup of vitality by CONNECTING WITH NATURE. Be mindful of internalised SELF-TALK.

CONSIDER

pursuing joy. Find what nourishes your energy and vitality. Laugh more, dance more, play more, connect more.

Adrenal Rebuilder Tincture: Formulas 1 and 2

HERBAL INGREDIENTS

Formula 1: Total depletion, low cortisol

¼ cup dried ashwagandha
   root
2 tablespoons dried
   rhodiola root
2 tablespoons dried
   licorice root
2 tablespoons dried
   tulsi leaf
2 tablespoons dried
   Siberian ginseng root

Formula 2: Frenetic depletion, high cortisol

½ cup dried ashwagandha
   root
¼ tablespoons dried oat
   straw or milky oat tops
¼ tablespoons dried
   passionflower leaf
¼ tablespoons dried
   tulsi leaf

When burnout is present – or there's even just a whispered hint of its impending presence – it is important to bring adaptogenic herbs on board, stat! There are two options with this tincture recipe. Formula 1 is most fitting for those who struggle to get out of bed in the morning and who labour to drum up any energy throughout their day – classically embodying a lower cortisol archetype. Formula 2 is for people who struggle to stay calm and sleep soundly, those who operate on a buzzy, frenetic energy although feeling totally depleted – classically embodying a higher cortisol archetype. Cortisol is a key steroid hormone intrinsically involved in the fight or flight response.

METHOD

Make the Tincture base recipe (p. 38) with the herbal ingredients.

DOSAGE

These tinctures need time to work. Weave them into your daily rhythms and give them at least 8–12 weeks of consistent compliance.

See Burnout Protocol (p. 48)
See also Endurance Support (p. 74)

The Awakener Caps

For downtrodden vitality and lacklustre energy. Working with this trio of adaptogenic plants encourages recalibration and a welcome return to vibrancy.

HERBAL INGREDIENTS

1 tablespoon licorice root powder

1 tablespoon ashwagandha root powder

1 tablespoon Siberian ginseng root powder

METHOD

Make the Capsules base recipe (p. 29) with the herbal ingredients.

DOSAGE

Weave these plant-powered capsules into your daily practice for at least 8–12 weeks to reap their rich medicinal bounty.

See Low Libido Protocol (p. 54)

Bright Eyes Tea

Many plant medicines are helpful for vision health. This delicious, piquant blend offers an antioxidant-rich profile laced within the eye-loving bilberry, working alongside the formidably named eyebright and co-star herbals to strengthen sparkly, bright eyes.

HERBAL INGREDIENTS

1 teaspoon dried eyebright leaf/stem/flowers

1 ½ teaspoons dried bilberries

1 teaspoon dried calendula petals

1 teaspoon dried cornflowers

2 teaspoons dried apple pieces

METHOD

Make the Medicinal Tea base recipe (p. 33) with the herbal ingredients.

See Longevity Protocol (p. 52)

The Dream Duster

HERBAL INGREDIENTS

1 tablespoon passionflower
  powder
1 tablespoon chamomile
  flower powder
1 tablespoon skullcap leaf
  powder

A gentle, plant-rich sedative blend to lull you into a receptive state of rest and a good night's sleep. You can keep this blend in powdered form and add into a liquid base, such as warmed plant mylk, with a touch of raw honey to soften the edges. But for the sake of your tastebuds – and accessible dosing – I suggest using capsules.

METHOD

Make the Capsules base recipe (p. 29) with the herbal ingredients.

DOSAGE

Best taken with dinner, allowing time for absorption and digestion pre-sleep.

See Insomnia/Poor Sleep Protocol (p. 50)
See also Menopause Protocol (p. 180)

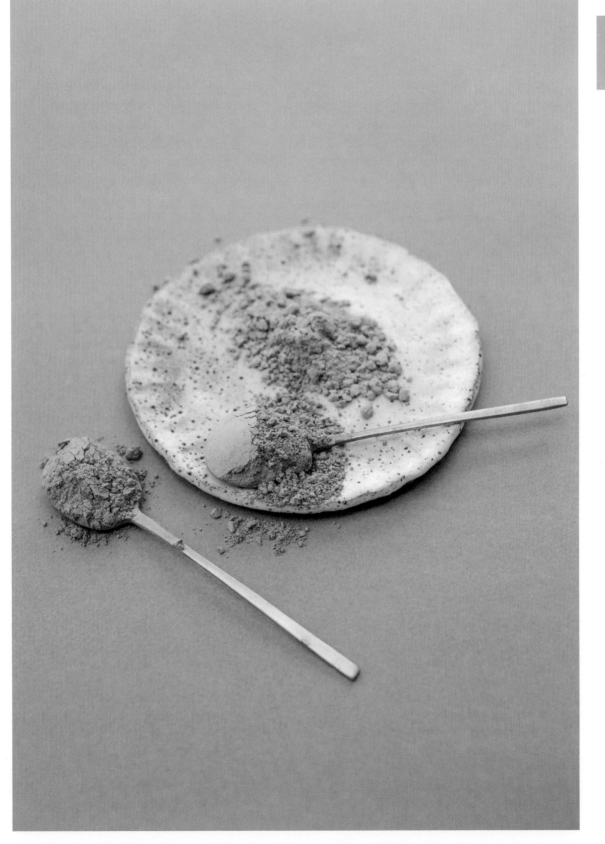

Iron-Lift Slow-Brew Syrup

For those in need of an iron-rich, nutritive boost. This mineral- and vitamin-dense brew is not only pleasant tasting, but also incredibly medicinal, with the medley of ingredients aiding the assimilation of iron and tonifying the blood. Keep this blend in the fridge to support and nourish your people, whatever their age!

HERBAL INGREDIENTS

6 tablespoons dried nettle leaf

4 tablespoons dried rosehips

2 tablespoons dried hibiscus flowers

2 tablespoons dried burdock root

3 tablespoons dried yellow dock root

4 tablespoons alfalfa leaf

3 tablespoons dried dandelion root

3 tablespoons dried hawthorn berries

2 tablespoons chlorella powder

METHOD

Make the Slow-Brew Syrup base recipe (p. 37) with the herbal ingredients.

DOSAGE

For sustained wellbeing, take a daily dose as outlined in the dosing guidelines (p. 45).

See Low Iron (p. 74)
See also Boosting Fertility Protocol (p. 176); Dysmenorrhoea (p. 208)

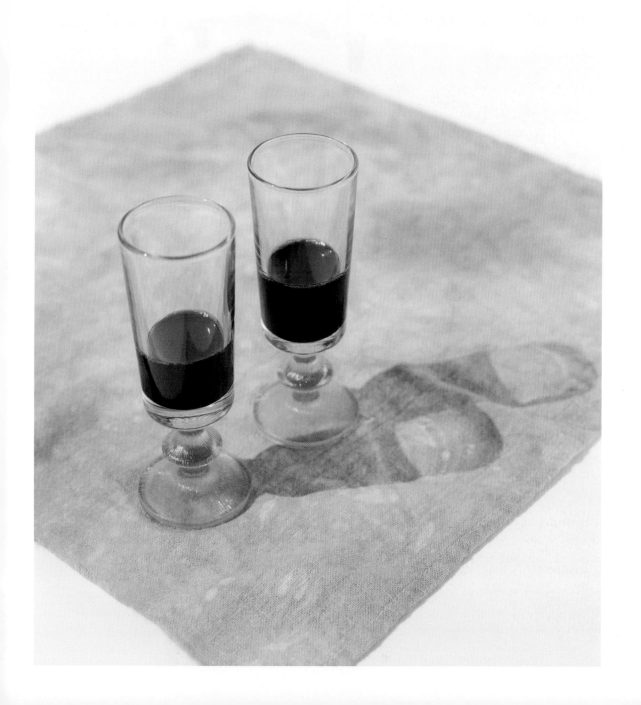

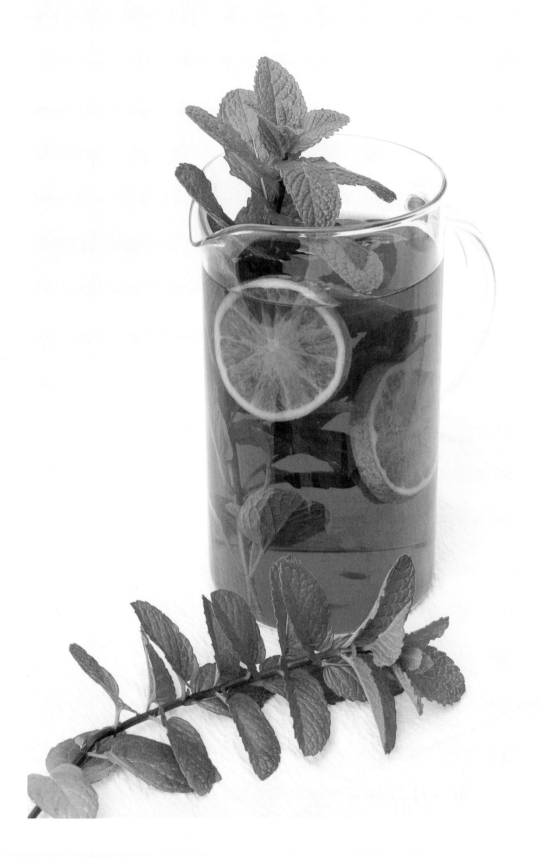

Live Long and Prosper

A cheerful, refreshing iced-tea 'mocktail', laden with acclaimed antioxidant-rich plants to promote wellbeing and longevity. Add citrus slices and fresh mint, sip in the sun and call it a day!

METHOD

Make the Medicinal Tea base recipe (p. 33) with the herbal ingredients. Cool and serve over ice.

See Longevity Protocol (p. 52)

HERBAL INGREDIENTS

1 teaspoon green tea
(swap to rooibos tea
if you are sensitive to
stimulants)

½ teaspoon dried hibiscus
flowers

1 teaspoon dried lemon
peel

½ teaspoon dried turmeric
rhizome

1 teaspoon dried goji
berries

The Lovers' Oxymel

A jammy aphrodisiac in a bottle! This delectable honey-based formula full of libido-enhancing and romancing herbs is perfect for when the flame of sensuality and embodied sexuality has dwindled. Most delicious taken straight on the tongue (or licked off the body of your favourite person).

HERBAL INGREDIENTS

½ cup dried schisandra
   berries
½ cup dried damiana leaf
1 cup dried rosehips
½ cup dried rose petals

METHOD

Make the Oxymel base recipe (p. 34) with the herbal ingredients.

See Low Libido Protocol (p. 54)

Lush Loins Tonic

A delicious milky tonic to fuel vitality and desire. Containing the medicinal mushroom cordyceps and hormone-harmonising maca root, this spicy chocolate milk–inspired blend can be served warm or over ice.

HERBAL INGREDIENTS

½ teaspoon cordyceps
   mushroom powder
1 tablespoon cacao or
   carob powder
½ teaspoon maca root
   powder
¼ teaspoon cinnamon
   powder
½ tablespoon lucuma
   powder
¼ teaspoon vanilla powder
1 teaspoon raw
   honey (optional, but
   recommended!)

METHOD

Make the Plant Mylk Tonic base recipe (p. 35) with the herbal ingredients.

See Low Libido Protocol (p. 54)
See also Endurance Support (p. 74)

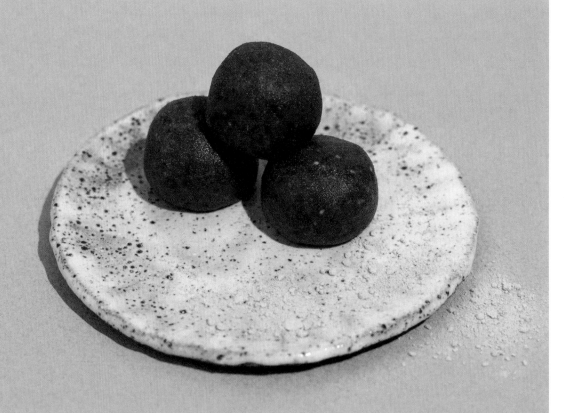

Maca Bliss Balls

HERBAL INGREDIENT

4 tablespoons maca root
  powder

NUTRITIONAL INGREDIENTS

3/4 cup almonds

3/4 cup walnuts

2 tablespoons chia seeds

1/2 cup Medjool dates

1–2 tablespoons hemp
  seeds

1 tablespoon sesame
  seeds

1–2 heaped tablespoons
  nut butter of choice

1–2 tablespoons carob
  powder

1–2 tablespoons coconut
  oil

Filled with the awesome maca, an adaptogenic root from the Andes, these bliss balls are super dense in nutrition, offering a dose of iron, iodine, potassium, calcium and more. Maca generously assists our ability to reshape the innate stress response and can be most helpful for poor vitality, offering a natural mood enhancement – particularly indicated for the symptoms of menopause, anxiety and depression. Maca root is a key libido enhancer and has an affinity for the reproductive organs, helping to boost fertility and support hormonal health. That said, these bliss balls are also a totally delicious energy-yielding snack.

MAKES UP TO 16 BLISS BALLS

METHOD

Place the almonds, walnuts and chia seeds in a food processor. Blend for 1 minute, until the nuts and seeds have been ground into a mealy flour.

Pit the dates and soften by soaking them in a bowl of warm water for 10 minutes. Drain the dates and pop them into the food processor along with all the other ingredients. Blitz for another minute until a dough forms.

Break off tablespoon-sized pieces of the dough and roll into balls. Keep them in a sealed container in the refrigerator for up to 7 days. Alternatively, you can freeze them – simply allow the balls to defrost for 10 or so minutes, to soften, then enjoy.

See Endurance Support (p. 74)
See also Boosting Fertility Protocol (p. 176); Depression Protocol (p. 274); Poor Focus/Cognition Protocol (p. 276)

Nettle and Oat Straw Infusion

A favourite of many herbalists, this is a deeply regenerative and restorative pairing. Working with this overnight infusion on a daily basis is unfussy and uncomplicated, and can have a profoundly nourishing impact. Rich in minerals and speaking fluently to both the nervous system and the adrenal system, this combo is one to bring on board when you are feeling weary and zapped. It has the added bonus of encouraging strong, lush hair.

HERBAL INGREDIENTS

2 tablespoons dried nettle leaf

2 tablespoons dried oat straw or milky oat tops

METHOD

Make the Overnight Water Infusion base recipe (p. 34) with the herbal ingredients.

DOSAGE

Work with this blend daily for at least 6 weeks to experience the positive impacts of the plants.

See Burnout Protocol (p. 48)
See also Postnatal Depletion Protocol (p. 216)

Nettle Tea

Nutritional, clearing, regenerative, blood-building and entirely versatile. Nettle tea is an outstanding herbal tea to befriend on the daily.

HERBAL INGREDIENT

2 teaspoons dried nettle leaf

METHOD

Make the Medicinal Tea base recipe (p. 33) or the Overnight Water Infusion base recipe (p. 34) with the nettle leaf.

See Low Iron (p. 74)

Slumber Drops

To assist a busy brain, overactive nervous system or wired body. Kava root and reishi mushroom lend their sleep magic, while rose calms and sweetens the spirit. These drops are wonderful if you need to reset sleep patterns, diffusing anxiety and ultimately allowing the body to regain equilibrium.

HERBAL INGREDIENTS

½ cup dried kava root
¼ cup dried reishi
½ cup dried rose petals

METHOD

Make the Glycetract Extract base recipe (p. 30) with the herbal ingredients.

DOSAGE

Best taken 30 minutes before sleep. Start with a lower dose to gauge receptivity to the blend, and work up to the dose recommended in the dosing guidelines (p. 45).

Please be mindful of keeping your maximum prolonged use of this blend to 1 month – kava should be taken only for short periods of time.

See Insomnia/Poor Sleep Protocol (p. 50)
See also Menopause Protocol (p. 180); Emotional Exhaustion (p. 292)

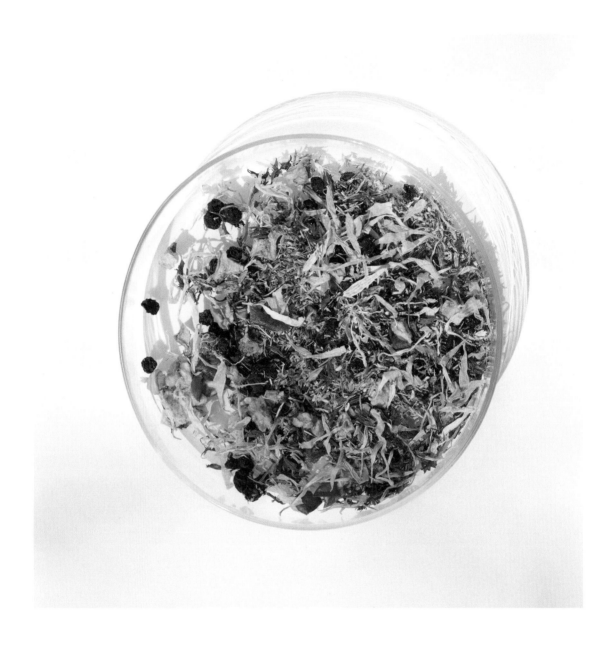

Bright Eyes Tea

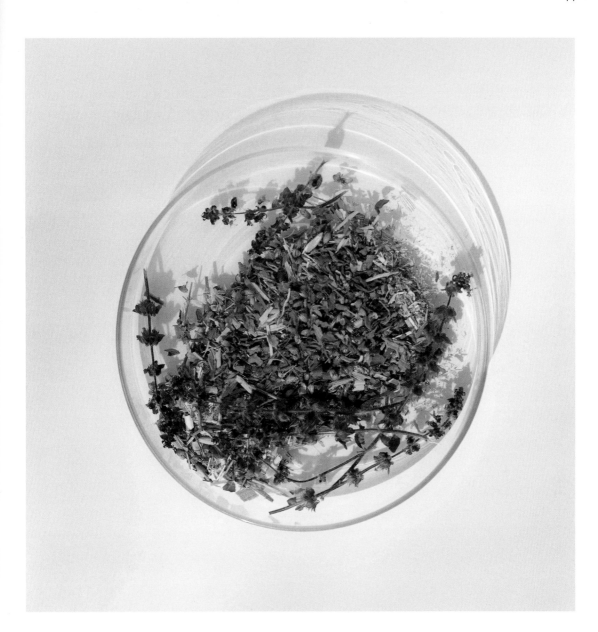

Zen Day Tea

Sustain Slow-Brew Syrup

HERBAL INGREDIENTS

2 tablespoons dried
   licorice root

3 tablespoons dried
   astragalus root

3 tablespoons dried
   ashwagandha root

4 slices dried reishi

4 tablespoons dried gotu
   kola

6 tablespoons dried oat
   straw or milky oat tops

4 tablespoons cinnamon
   chips

¼ cup goji berries

A sweet, syrupy chorus of revival! This is a wonderfully supportive treacle to replenish the body, infused with adaptogenic and nourishing herbs aplenty. Particularly helpful for those with depleted energy, this robust blend works to reconstruct innate vitality and counteract the adverse impacts of stress and exhaustion.

METHOD

Make the Slow-Brew Syrup base recipe (p. 37) with the herbal ingredients.

See Low Energy (p. 74)

Timelessness Tincture

This is a potent tincture for neurological health, with plants for focus, plants for memory and plants for graceful ageing. Bring this omnipotent mixed quintet of adaptogens and keen mind encouragers on board when concentration is dwindling or memory recall is fuzzy.

HERBAL INGREDIENTS

½ cup dried gingko leaf
½ cup dried gynostemma
   leaf
½ cup dried brahmi leaf
½ cup dried tulsi flowers/
   leaf
½ cup dried gotu kola leaf

METHOD

Make the Tincture base recipe (p. 38) with the herbal ingredients.

DOSAGE

Work with this blend for at least 8 weeks for sustained and notable impact.

See Longevity Protocol (p. 52)
See also Poor Focus/Cognition Protocol (p. 276)

Zen Day Tea

Super simple, super zen. Tulsi tastes like heaven, and the oat straw/milky oat tops nourish deeply – together, they're a perfect pair to support the nervous system, combat anxiety and counter a hyper-stress response.

HERBAL INGREDIENTS

3 teaspoons dried tulsi
   leaf/flowers
2 teaspoons dried oat
   straw or milky oat tops

METHOD

Make the Medicinal Tea base recipe (p. 33) or the Overnight Water Infusion base recipe (p. 34) with the herbal ingredients.

See Insomnia/Poor Sleep Protocol (p. 50)

Rescue Remedies

ENDURANCE SUPPORT

For athletes in particular, endurance is a big deal. Maca, turmeric, Siberian ginseng, cordyceps, American ginseng, ashwagandha and rhodiola are all indicated here. To weave in these esteemed herbals, give one or a combination of these recipes a go: **Maca Bliss Balls** (p. 67), **The Golden One** tonic (p. 130), the **Lush Loins Tonic** (p. 65) or the **Adrenal Rebuilder Tincture: Formulas 1 and 2** (p. 56).

LOW ENERGY

When you are not quite burnt out, but know you are tired, with your energy waning throughout the day, it is time to bring on all the nourishing adaptogenic and vitality-catalysing plant medicines. One of the most effective is the **Sustain Slow-Brew Syrup** (p. 72), a daily dose of a harmoniously jumbled, plant-rich syrup that is not only delectable but also truly energy-boosting. Rich in vitamins and minerals, adaptogens, longevity enhancers and nervines, this is a mix to keep on hand.

PS: Check out the Burnout Protocol (p. 48) for deeper guidance on rebalancing your energy stores.

LOW IRON

Particularly common in menstruating people, low blood-iron levels can be an underlying cause of poor vitality. Fatigue, malaise, a sallow complexion, chest pain, breathlessness, anxiety, foggy brain, poor focus, exhaustion when exercising and dizziness can all be involved with low iron levels. Combat symptoms by taking a daily dose of the **Iron-Lift Slow-Brew Syrup** (p. 60) a quite delicious medicinal plant-rich preparation full of iron-giving herbs. Sipping on the blood-building **Nettle Tea** (p. 68) throughout the day is highly recommended.

PS: These iron-rich herbal prescriptions can be most supportive and will bolster an increase in iron intake. But before adding in supplementation, it's best to have a full iron-studies blood test via your medical provider to be certain of low levels.

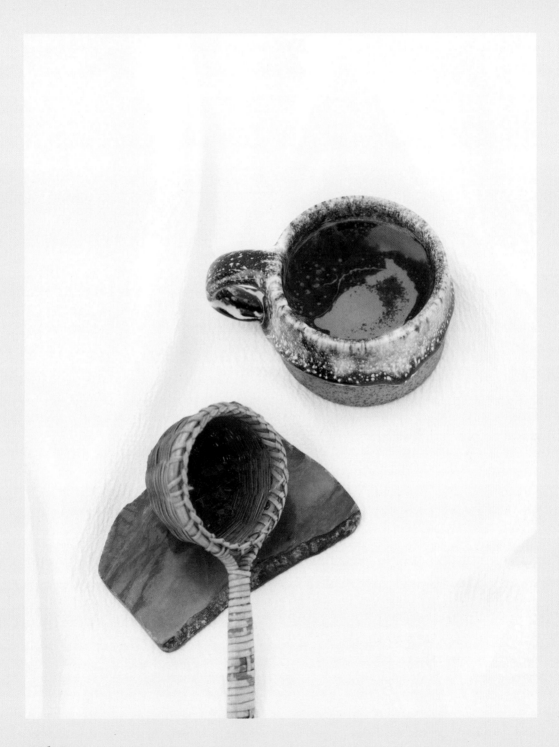

Nettle Tea

Immunity

The immune system is a master neutraliser of free radicals, as well as potentially harmful exogenous (environmental) elements and endogenous (internal) cellular changes. The primary role knitted throughout the hyper-intelligent framework of the immune system is to create barriers against pathogens (viruses, bacteria, fungi and parasites) that could potentially weaken your body and bring about illness. Immunity is a network of intrinsic complexity – not representing one single system per se but, rather, an interconnected gamut of cell, tissue, protein and organ involvement.

A perfect duet of words describes the two systems existing under the immune system umbrella: the innate (non-specific) immune system and the adaptive (specific) immune system responses. The innate and adaptive subsystems create a call and response, and work in an alliance to protect, preserve and adapt, in order to guard against possible disharmony.

Ultimately, the immune system is the defender, the warrior on the front lines.

Stress inhibits the fundamental functioning of the immune system. When we are stressed, we are commonly more susceptible to colds, cold sores, mouth ulcers and so on. So, what can we do to activate immunity? We can welcome in the Pillars to Thrive (p. 16), with a big emphasis on rest, drinking lots of water and eating nutritious food to fortify our innate and adaptive immune abilities.

And we can bring on the plant medicines from nature, those remedies that enhance and encourage our intrinsic immunity.

From colds, to convalescing, what follows is a representation of how the plants may assist you and your immune system.

Consider these the keys to supporting your immune system

— There's a reason that there are traditions around the world based on eating warm foods when ill – gently cooked, super-nourishing foods restore the fire within your body, bringing energy back to your system and aiding recovery. Cold foods and drinks can be a little jarring on the body and really are best avoided for any immune-building health endeavours. So, say hello to stews, curries, hotpots and herbal teas.

— The immune system will greatly appreciate a squeaky-clean diet full of wholesome foods. An alcohol-free period, as well as low-to-zero caffeine intake and removal of sugar from the diet (although a little honey to soothe the throat is A-OK – it holds medicinal qualities that refined sugars do not), will seriously aid your recovery.

— Up your vitamin C intake! It's an essential micronutrient and water-soluble antioxidant that helps bolster our immune system. A little heads-up: although we generally want to avoid raw foods when restoring a depressed immune system, cooking reduces vitamin C content, so consider adding raw C-rich foods to your meals or drinking vitamin C–dense plant and herb smoothies. Fortunately, dried lemon and orange peel make beautiful vitamin C–rich additions to any herbal teas and syrups!

Foods super rich in vitamin C

— Broccoli
— Brussels sprouts
— Cauliflower
— Citrus fruits
— Dandelion leaves
— Guava
— Kale
— Kiwifruit
— Papaya
— Pineapple
— Red capsicum (red pepper)
— Rockmelon (cantaloupe)
— Sorrel
— Strawberries
— Tomatoes

Herbs super rich in vitamin C

— Elderberries
— Hibiscus
— Lemongrass
— Nasturtium leaves and flowers (best fresh)
— Nettle leaf
— Pine/Spruce/Fir needles (best fresh)
— Rosehips
— Thyme

DAILY PROTOCOL

Acute Colds

Morning	Throughout the Day	
RINSE with a **Neti Pot Sinus Rinse** (p. 115). Containing olive leaf, mullein, chamomile and ribwort, this rinse will alleviate nasal congestion and open airways. Once you have prepared the sinus rinse, utilise the whole pot. **DRINK** a radical, herbal-rich, germ-busting **Cannonball Shot** (p. 95) to kick-start and flush the body. Remember, the more 'kick' in the flavour, the better!	**DRINK** a pot of **The Garden of Immuni-Tea** (p. 103), made with thyme, oregano, lemon and manuka honey. This low-maintenance mix holds wonderful antiviral and antibacterial elements. **EAT** **Cold-Buster Candies** (p. 100). Containing elderberry, mullein, marshmallow and echinacea, they will soothe the throat and reinforce your inner immune defence.	
Enhancements	**CONSIDER** adding in the **Acute Andrographis and Echinacea Tincture** (p. 90) if you are at the very beginning of acute cold symptoms, and follow the acute dose suggestions.	

Here is a robust plan to protect, fortify and enhance the innate immune response within – a perfect protocol to action when you feel a scratchy sore throat or the sniffles creeping in. Most wonderful when you feel a little run-down or are weathering the seasonal changes. When you feel a cold looming, it's best to really go in strong and flush your body with all the plant protectors.

	Afternoon	Evening
	DRINK	**SOAK**
	a **Chagacino** (p. 96), to re-stoke the warmth within. Made with chaga, this potent, medicinal, mushroom-rich concoction is the perfect afternoon pick-me-up for the immune system – with the added bonus of being totally delicious.	in a bath imbued with a **Ginger Bath Bomb** (p. 106), to activate your lymphatic system and sweat the germs out.
		SLEEP
		with some **Garlic in Your Socks** (p. 103) – an overnight self-defensive act undertaken through the absorption channels of your feet.

PRACTISE THE PILLARS

HYDRATION is key in shifting a virus or bacterial infection. **REST** is the deepest, most effective medicine, allowing your body to heal and recover with ease.

Chest Cold

Morning, Afternoon and Evening	Throughout the Day
### SPOON the **Lung Love Syrup** (p. 113), a deliciously infused demulcent and gently expectorant syrup, to target the chest. ### POP 2 **Grand Garlic Capsules** (p. 107) with every main meal, totalling 6 capsules daily with meals. Garlic is majorly effective against infections and is a most wonderful mucus-mover for the lungs.	### DRINK a double-strength cup of **The Garden of Immuni-Tea** (p. 103) with a spoonful of added manuka honey. This antiviral and antibacterial herbal brew offers decongestant properties and immune stimulation. In an active infection, aim for 3–6 cups over the course of the day. ### DOSE UP on a shot of 5–10 millilitres (1–2 teaspoons) of **Nasturtium Flower Vinegar** (p. 114) mixed in a little warm water. This ridiculously pretty ruby-red infused floral vinegar packs a mega punch for a chest infection or chest cold. Aim to do this at least twice daily when symptoms are present. Be brave, be bold!

A cold or flu will commonly make its way into the chest, and a respiratory tract infection may set in. It is super important to boost immunity and target the chest with herbals that are fluent in lung support, while also offering medicinal plants that are antibacterial and antiviral in nature to prevent or reduce infection.

Enhancements

PRACTISE THE PILLARS

HYDRATE – warm liquids all the way. **REST;** really, really rest up. Allow yourself time off from intensive body movement. Be sure to **CONNECT WITH NATURE,** get some sunshine on the skin. **GOOD FOOD** only.

EAT

all the vitamin C–rich foods that come your way! Wherever possible, weave onions and garlic into your meals. Consider cooked, warming foods such as **Scrap Broth** (p. 121), congee and soups galore.

DAILY PROTOCOL

Chronic Low Immunity

Morning and Evening	Throughout the Day
### SPOON a tablespoon dose of the **The Orange Orchard Oxymel** (p. 116). This very yum yet very medicinal plant preparation is full of orange peel and rosehips, both excellent sources of vitamin C, while elderflower and echinacea offer poignant immune support – all infused in a base of raw honey and apple cider vinegar. ### POP 2 capsules of the **Supreme Shrooms** (p. 121). Taken twice daily with meals, these powdered medicinal mushrooms offer impactful immune support. The powdered medicinal reishi, maitake, chaga, cordyceps and turkey tail mushrooms weave a field of fungi-rich synergy.	### DRINK a constantly renewed pot of **Anchor of Immunity Tea** (p. 91), to fortify immunity. This hardy simmered decoction contains licorice root, astragalus root, schisandra berries and Siberian ginseng root, a quartet of herbs that not only lifts a downtrodden immune system but also gently supports the liver. All while offering the adrenal system a helpful boost in combating fatigue and the impacts of stress. ### SIP a cup of **Scrap Broth** (p. 119), infused with astragalus, turmeric, reishi and shiitake mushrooms, garlic and onions. This nutrient-dense liquid gold offers deep immune support to rebuild and restore. To add an extra kick, pour in a dose of **Cannonball Shot** (p. 95).

If you are constantly becoming ill, catching every virus or bug that crosses your path, regard this as a perfect opportunity to offer the immune system extra support. These herbal interventions have a wonderful way of supporting a downtrodden immune system and are particularly effective in regenerating innate immune defence. This protocol also offers poignant tips to help you out of a postviral slump. Use for at least 4 weeks.

Enhancements

PRACTISE THE PILLARS

Allow yourself to **REST** when you are feeling run-down. Adjust your **BODY MOVEMENT** and exercise far less intensively when your energy stores are lower. Stay **HYDRATED**. Focus on nourishing your body with **GOOD FOOD**.

CONSIDER

temperature as a remedy! Stay warm, eat warm foods, drink warm liquids. Warmth is extremely supportive as you rebuild a depleted body and being.

Dry Cough

Persistent dry coughs are the pits. They cause throat irritation and require repetitive effort from the body – all without any phlegm yield. In addition to creating a red, raw throat, an unproductive dry cough can keep you up at night. It is important to regularly soothe and moisten the respiratory passages to combat any tickles and dryness.

Morning and Evening	Throughout the Day
DOSE UP on a **Cannonball Shot** (p. 95), to warm the insides and shake up immunity. **GARGLE** on a preparation of the **Sage and Saltwater Gargle** (p. 117) – basically a strong sage tea infusion with the addition of sea salt. This gargle is most effective when used after meals.	**SPRAY** the **Botanical Throat Spray** (p. 91), aimed at the back of the throat. This tasty blend will soothe rawness and herbally coat the irritated throat surface. **SPOON** the **Cough Relief Syrup** (p. 100), to quell persistent coughing. Mullein, ribwort, fennel, licorice, wild cherry bark and horehound unite to promote ease for the respiratory passages and calm a weary throat. When the cough is acute, take hourly or as needed.

Enhancements	PRACTISE THE PILLARS **HYDRATE** aplenty – warm liquids are far better than colder liquids. **REST** up. EAT slippery soft foods. Warming **Scrap Broth** (p. 119) would be wonderful, or try the **Slippery Elm Paste** (p. 231) stirred into porridge.

DAILY PROTOCOL

Hay Fever

'Allergies' can mean many things. You could have seasonal allergies, or allergies to an animal. This protocol is most helpful for the symptoms of hay fever (allergic rhinitis): a stuffed-up or runny nose, itchy eyes and throat, and repeated sneezing.

Morning and Evening	Throughout the Day
DOSE UP on the **Allergy-Ease Tincture** (p. 90), full of herbals to impact an overactive histamine response, bringing calmness and stability. **RINSE** and flush nasal passageways with the herbal-infused **Neti Pot Sinus Rinse** (p. 115).	**DRINK** from a water bottle filled with a heaped teaspoon of **C Powder** (p. 92), for a tart, plant-rich burst of vitamin C. Vitamin C is a key player in allergy-response reduction. Citrus peel, hibiscus, rosehips and strawberry powder create a pretty pink cordial-like base for you to sip on, and you can add a sweet (optional) dollop of **Nettle, Reishi and Rose Raw Honey** (p. 115).

Enhancements

PRACTISE THE PILLARS

Focus on **HYDRATION** aplenty. Nourish your body with **GOOD FOOD**.

CONSIDER

supplementation with extra vitamin C and quercetin. It really can be helpful in calming a hay-fever storm. Weave fresh ginger, garlic, onions, horseradish and cayenne into your meals whenever possible. These five seriously potent plants will assist in unblocking any sinus congestion and promoting nasal clearance. Many plants are rich in quercetin, a powerhouse bioflavonoid, key for the treatment of allergies. Try the **Cannonball Shot** (p. 95)!

Influenza

Morning, Afternoon and Evening	Throughout the Day
POP a combination of 2 medicinal, mushroom-dense **Supreme Shrooms** capsules (p. 121) and 2 **Flu-Buster Capsules** (p. 102), containing yarrow, elderflower, boneset and thyme to support the body and shoo out any invaders. Take these with a full meal, three times daily. **DOSE UP** on a shot of **Nasturtium Flower Vinegar** (p. 114) mixed in a little warm water. This traditional folk remedy offers an intense, immune-defensive kick.	**SIP** on a cup or three of **Scrap Broth** (p. 119). This broth is laden with onions, garlic, shiitake and turmeric to enhance immunity. It is super helpful to keep pre-made batches of this warming brew in the freezer to be defrosted when needed. **DRINK** a steady supply of **Immune Enhancer Tea** (p. 113), a blended herbal mishmash containing echinacea and elderberries, which are rich in vitamin C. **FUMIGATE** the house with **Herbal Fumigation** (p. 110), a steamy, aromatic rapid-boil to clear the air of germs. Rosemary, sage, eucalyptus and thyme are all indicated here.

Much like an acute cold – but with the added severity of fevers, chills, body aches and headaches – a flu can be intense to weather. Influenza will often lead to secondary infections such as bronchitis, so it is important to get in there swiftly with herbal support, to assist the body systems to clear the bugs and encourage an uncomplicated recovery. The flu calls for stillness, rest, and lots and lots of hydration.

Enhancements

PRACTISE THE PILLARS

REST is non-negotiable: it is the most important element in shifting an active influenza. **HYDRATION** is key – focus on warm liquids galore.

CONSIDER

the recipes in the Immunity section; honestly, any of them would be helpful. If you have a sore throat, use the **Coat Your Throat Tea** (p. 97) or the **Botanical Throat Spray** (p. 91).

DAILY PROTOCOL

Sinus

Plant medicines are an underrated prescription for sinus issues, whether it be sinus congestion, sinus headaches or sinus infections. Simple interventions, such as herbal steams and rinses, make a world of difference in clearing up uncomfortable symptoms.

Morning and Evening	Throughout the Day
### RINSE with a **Neti Pot Sinus Rinse** (p. 115), to flush the sinuses and encourage decongestion with an aromatic edge. Olive leaf, mullein, chamomile and ribwort all come on board to assist. *or* ### INHALE the **Heroic Herbal Steam Bowl** (p. 112), with its antimicrobial, antibacterial powers. Made with aromatic plants, such as oregano and thyme, it moisturises airways and decongests.	### SPOON **Onion and Garlic Honey** (p. 116) onto your tongue, to support immunity and clear congestion. Although this sounds thoroughly unappetising, it is honestly not that bad! Using raw honey as the base really softens the culinary flavours and adds an extra medicinal element. ### DRINK **Clear Passage Tea** (p. 96), full of immune-supportive and sinus-specific plants.

Enhancements	PRACTISE THE PILLARS **HYDRATE** aplenty. **REST** aplenty. EAT potent foods to clear your sinus passages. Chilli, wasabi, horseradish, garlic, onions, ginger and nasturtiums are all mucolytic plant heroes.

DAILY PROTOCOL

Wet Cough

We want to encourage the lungs to expel any congestion or infection, so if you have a wet, phlegmy cough this is a positive thing – mostly! However, when it becomes tiresome and overly persistent, there are ways to ease and dissipate a wet cough with support from our plants in arms.

Morning and Evening	Throughout the Day
### SPOON the **Lung Love Syrup** (p. 113), to assist in shifting mucus and calming bronchial passageways. With thyme, rosehips, elderberries, elecampane, mullein and marshmallow, this tasty syrup offers a wealth of nourishment for a persistent wet cough. ### POP the **Grand Garlic Capsules** (p. 107), for added antibacterial power and immunity enhancement.	### DRINK **Calm Chest Tea** (p. 92), a full-flavoured formulation that eases persistent coughing and encourages the break-up of phlegm. ### STEAM your respiratory passageways to ameliorate and clear congestion multiple times daily. Before jumping into a warming shower, pop a few drops of rosemary essential oil onto the shower floor – the aromatic steam build-up eases respiratory irritation. Or make a **Heroic Herbal Steam Bowl** (p. 112), with fresh rosemary or eucalyptus leaves.
Enhancements	**PRACTISE THE PILLARS** Stay well **HYDRATED** – warm liquids over cold all the way! Claim **REST** when possible. Eat really **GOOD FOOD**, focusing on warm foods and adding generous amounts of onions and garlic to your cooking. Reduce the intensity of **BODY MOVEMENT** – gentle movement is best.

Acute Andrographis and Echinacea Tincture

The perfect tincture to boost low immunity and help you sidestep the impending clutches of that 'under the weather' feeling. Best taken at the first signs of any cold- or flu-like symptoms, this potent combination is a wonderful tincture to have on hand in your home dispensary.

HERBAL INGREDIENTS

½ cup dried andrographis
   leaf
½ cup dried echinacea
   leaf/stem/flowers/root
2 tablespoons dried ginger
   rhizome

METHOD

Make the Tincture base recipe (p. 38) with the herbal ingredients.

DOSAGE

If symptoms are acute, be sure to dose accordingly, as suggested in the dosing guidelines (p. 45).

See Acute Colds Protocol (p. 78)

Allergy-Ease Tincture

When allergies are present and persistent, work closely with this quartet of allergy-specific supporters to calm down the reactive storm of seasonal or environmental hay fever.

HERBAL INGREDIENTS

½ cup dried nettle leaf
½ cup albizia bark
½ cup elderflower
½ cup goldenrod
   flowers/leaf

METHOD

Make the Tincture base recipe (p. 38) with the herbal ingredients.

DOSAGE

For a marked impact, pre-empt the onset of allergies if possible. Start taking this tincture daily, at the everyday dose suggested in the dosing guidelines (p. 45).

See Hay Fever Protocol (p. 85)

Anchor of Immunity Tea

A root-rich, slow-simmered decoction, this blend is fitting for those overcoming a bout of low immunity or niggling post-viral symptoms, or just for general convalescence. Adaptogenic in nature, this formula is also the perfect restorative tea to combat the internal impacts of stress, working to build resilience while raising innate vitality and reinstating wellness.

HERBAL INGREDIENTS

½ teaspoon dried licorice root

1 teaspoon dried astragalus root

1 teaspoon dried schisandra berries

1 teaspoon dried Siberian ginseng root

METHOD

Make the Decoction base recipe (p. 29) with the herbal ingredients.

See Chronic Low Immunity Protocol (p. 82)

Botanical Throat Spray

At the onset of any signs of a sore throat, spray frequently. With antimicrobial forces, immune boosters and soothing elements, this easy-on-the-tastebuds blend will keep the throat protected and on guard.

HERBAL INGREDIENTS

2 teaspoons dried echinacea root

3 teaspoons dried marshmallow root

2 teaspoons dried elderberries

1 teaspoon dried licorice root

3 teaspoons of dried whole cloves

4 teaspoons dried sage

1 teaspoon raw honey or manuka honey

METHOD

Make the Decoction base recipe (p. 29) with the herbal ingredients, adjusting the amount of water in the base recipe to 2 cups to yield a smaller amount of medicinal brew. Add the honey to the finished decoction and decant into a small spray bottle.

DOSAGE

If you are experiencing sore throat symptoms, really amp up the dosage every 1–2 hours, following the dosing guidelines (p. 45).

See Dry Cough Protocol (p. 84); Influenza Protocol (p. 86)

C Powder

An emboldened, whole-plant vitamin C powder. Offering a beneficial bounty of plants rich in antioxidants and vitamin C, it has a sour-sweet tang on the palate. Utilise for immunity aplenty – and radiant skin! It can be added as a smoothie booster or stirred vigorously into water for a pink-hued plant cordial.

HERBAL INGREDIENTS

3 tablespoons hibiscus
  powder
3 tablespoons rosehip
  powder
1 tablespoon lemon peel
  powder
1 tablespoon orange peel
  powder
4 tablespoons strawberry
  powder

METHOD

Make the Herbal Powder base recipe (p. 33) with the herbal ingredients.

See Hay Fever Protocol (p. 85)
See also Shingles (p. 268)

Calm Chest Tea

A richly supportive blend to alleviate a burdened upper respiratory system. Keep on hand as a remedy for a cough, cold or sore throat, and sip on cups throughout the day when you feel the call to weave in extra support.

HERBAL INGREDIENTS

3 teaspoons dried aniseed
1 teaspoon dried hyssop
  flowers/leaf
1 teaspoon dried mullein
  leaf
1 teaspoon dried ribwort
  leaf
1 teaspoon dried sage
1 teaspoon dried rosehip
  shells

METHOD

Make the Medicinal Tea base recipe (p. 33) with the herbal ingredients.

See Wet Cough Protocol (p. 89)
See also Sore Throat (p. 123)

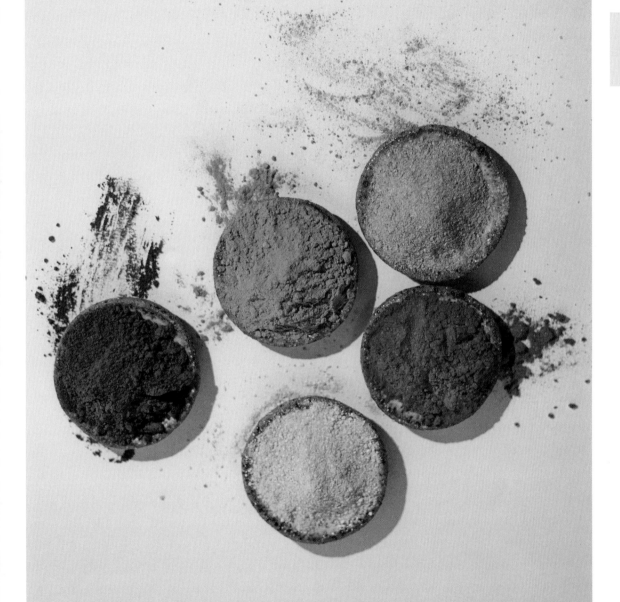

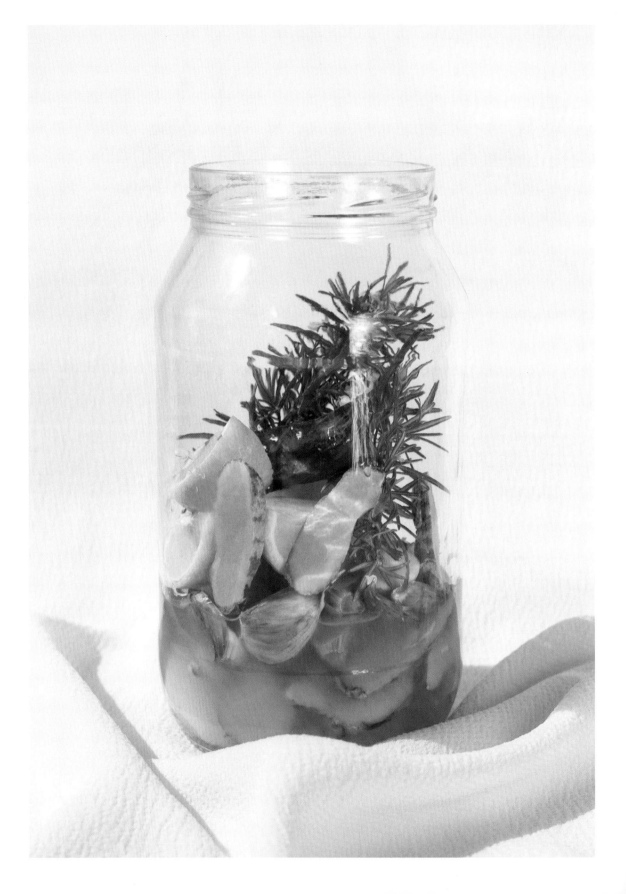

Cannonball Shot

HERBAL INGREDIENTS

½ cup finely chopped
   fresh ginger rhizome
12 cloves garlic, minced
2 tablespoons finely
   chopped fresh turmeric
   rhizome or 1 tablespoon
   turmeric rhizome powder
1 large onion, chopped
¼ cup grated fresh
   horseradish
1 lemon, sliced thinly
4 fresh rosemary sprigs
   or 2 tablespoons dried
   rosemary
½ cup raw honey
½ teaspoon dried cayenne
   powder
1–2 fresh chillies, chopped
   (omit if you are heat
   sensitive!)

This heat-infused vinegar pays homage to the herbal legend 'fire cider', full of common kitchen ingredients that work to support immunity. So easy to make, yielding a healthful bounty that can be used to douse salads and veggies, as a base for dressings or in everyday cooking. It can be diluted with water or taken neat as a ballsy shot to activate and strengthen the immune system.

IMMUNITY

METHOD

Make the Vinegar base recipe (p. 39) with the herbal ingredients.

See Acute Colds Protocol (p. 78); Chronic Low Immunity Protocol (p. 82); Dry Cough Protocol (p. 84)

Chagacino

This medicinal mushroom–laced tonic is emboldened with the powers of immune-stimulating chaga, held within the grounding base of dandelion and maca. And it tastes straight-up delicious! Truly perfect drunk warmed, or iced, on the daily.

HERBAL INGREDIENTS

1–2 teaspoons dandelion
   root powder
½ teaspoon chaga powder
½ teaspoon maca powder
¼ teaspoon mesquite
   powder
a pinch of sea salt
a touch of raw honey
   (optional)

METHOD

Make the Plant Mylk Tonic base recipe (p. 35) with the herbal ingredients.

See Acute Colds Protocol (p. 78)

Clear Passage Tea

A sinus-specific blend to alleviate nasal congestion and encourage free-flowing passages. This blend works to rouse immunity and subdue underlying allergies and inflammation.

METHOD

Make the Medicinal Tea base recipe (p. 33) with the herbal ingredients.

HERBAL INGREDIENTS

2 teaspoons dried
   elderflower
1 teaspoon dried
   calendula petals
4 teaspoons dried ginger
   rhizome
1 teaspoon dried
   goldenrod flowers/leaf
1 teaspoon dried eyebright
   leaf/stem/flowers

DOSAGE

When symptoms are present, aim for the higher end of the acute dose suggested in the dosing guidelines (p. 44).

See Sinus Protocol (p. 88)

Clove Oil

The mighty clove, rich in volatile oils and antiseptic in nature, is a consistent ally in treating all things toothache and gum-pain related. Clove oil is exceptionally easy to make and super handy to have in your home apothecary. Simply dab onto the gum or tooth in question for a gentle numbing sensation. This can be most helpful for a teething bub or grumpy grown-up weathering discomfort.

IMMUNITY

HERBAL INGREDIENT

1 cup dried whole cloves

METHOD

Make the Herbal-Infused Oil base recipe (p. 31) with the cloves.

See Mouth Ulcers/Canker Sores (p. 123)
See also Teething (p. 233); Toothache (p. 303)

Coat Your Throat Tea

A demulcent blend to relieve a sore throat, with the analgesic benefits of clove and the soothing sensation of licorice and marshmallow to ease rawness and irritation.

METHOD

Make the Medicinal Tea base recipe (p. 33) with the herbal ingredients.

See Influenza Protocol (p. 86)
See also Sore Throat (p. 123)

HERBAL INGREDIENTS

½ teaspoon dried licorice root
2 teaspoons dried linden flowers
3 ½ teaspoons dried marshmallow root
10 dried whole cloves or ¼ teaspoon clove powder

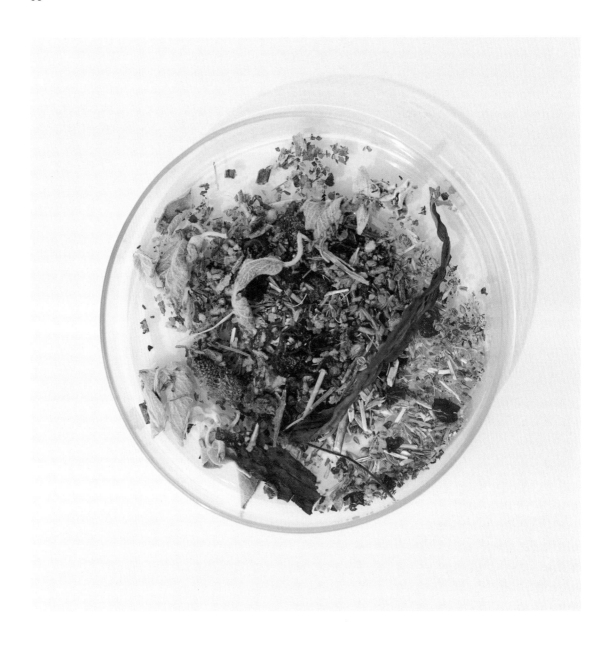

Calm Chest Tea

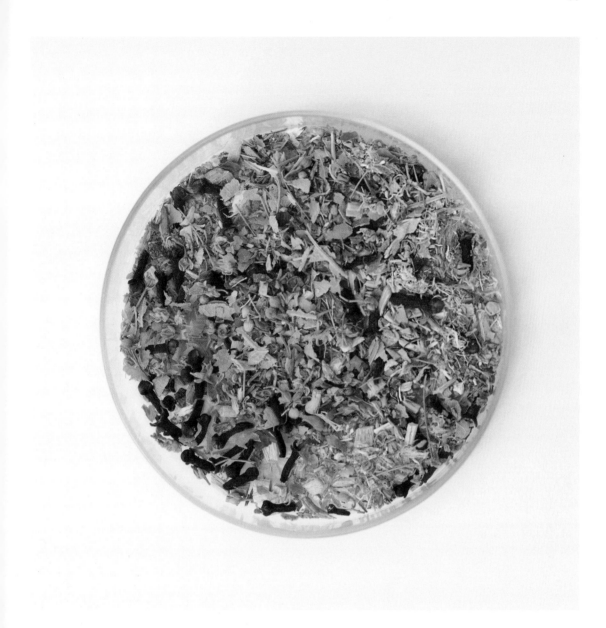

Coat Your Throat Tea

Cold-Buster Candies

Ideal for a dry, irritated, sore throat or chest congestion. With a tasty elderberry tang, these candies bypass the use of refined sugar – unlike most packaged herbal sore-throat suckers. Convincingly yum for children or those with sensitive palates.

HERBAL INGREDIENTS

2 teaspoons dried
    echinacea root/leaf/
    flowers
3 teaspoons dried
    elderberries
2 teaspoons dried
    marshmallow root
2 teaspoons dried
    mullein leaf

METHOD

Make the Candies base recipe (p. 28) with the herbal ingredients.

See Acute Colds Protocol (p. 78)

Cough Relief Syrup

A lubricator of the lungs! Bring this syrup on board to pacify the passages and quell a repetitive dry, unproductive cough or a tickle in the chest. A great syrup to have on hand in the cooler seasons, for the little ones as well as the grown-up ones!

HERBAL INGREDIENTS

3 tablespoons dried
    mullein leaf
2 tablespoons dried
    ribwort leaf
2 tablespoons dried fennel
    seeds
1 tablespoon dried licorice
    root
2 tablespoons dried wild
    cherry bark
2 tablespoons dried
    horehound
2 tablespoons dried lemon
    peel
1 tablespoon dried
    cinnamon bark

METHOD

Make the Simple Syrup base recipe (p. 37) with the herbal ingredients.

See Dry Cough Protocol (p. 84)

Ease the Eyes Wash

HERBAL INGREDIENTS

1 teaspoon dried eyebright
  leaf/stem/flowers
1 teaspoon dried calendula
  flowers
1 teaspoon dried
  chamomile flowers

Use this easy-to-prep wash and compress to combat and clear a bacterial eye infection, such as conjunctivitis.

METHOD

Make the Wash base recipe (p. 39) with the herbal ingredients. Simply dip a clean face washer or cotton pad into the warm wash, hold the pad over the eye to soften and clear the hardened discharge, then wipe it away gently.

See Conjunctivitis (p. 122)

Echinacea Tincture

HERBAL INGREDIENT

¾ cup dried echinacea
  root

An essential tincture to have on hand in any home herbal kit! Echinacea stimulates both the lymphatic and immune systems, a perfect pair of actions to counteract immune and skin-health imbalances. In tincture form, the potency of this stellar herb is strong and accessible. Use this remedy to support immunity, to shorten the severity and duration of colds, flus and upper respiratory tract concerns, to stimulate the lymphatic system and assist with skin complaints, to defend a looming UTI – and much more. Those sensitive to alcohol can make a glycerin version with ease.

METHOD

Make the Tincture base recipe (p. 38) or the Glycetract Extract base recipe (p. 30) with the echinacea.

DOSAGE

At the onset of any cold-like symptoms, reach for this tincture stat and follow the acute dosage suggestions given in the dosing guidelines (p. 44–45).

See Warts (p. 123)
See also Fortified Pregnancy Support – For Immunity (p. 212);
Mastitis (p. 232)

Fever Tea

When a fever is present, this blend will help trigger the innate mechanisms that allow your body to sweat the fever out and normalise body temperature. This is also an entirely appropriate all-round prescription for colds and flus, headaches and catarrh.

HERBAL INGREDIENTS

1 teaspoon dried feverfew
    flowers/leaf
1 teaspoon dried
    elderflower
½ teaspoon dried
    peppermint leaf
½ teaspoon dried yarrow
    flowers/leaf
½ teaspoon dried mallow
    flowers

METHOD

Make the Medicinal Tea base recipe (p. 33) with the herbal ingredients.

DOSAGE

It is important to utilise this tea frequently to support treatment of an active fever. Follow the acute dosing guidelines (p. 44).

See Chickenpox (p. 122); Fever (p. 122)

Flu-Buster Capsules

This formula is best utilised when symptoms indicate that you are at the early or acute stage of a flu: looming fevers, chills and body aches; blocked sinuses; a sore throat; and a tiresome cough. Please be sure to use boneset (*Eupatorium perfoliatum*) and not comfrey (or knitbone, *Symphytum officinale*), as the two are often confused.

HERBAL INGREDIENTS

½ tablespoon dried yarrow
    flowers/leaf
1 tablespoon dried
    elderflower
½ tablespoon dried
    boneset flowers/leaf
1 tablespoon dried thyme

METHOD

Make the Capsules base recipe (p. 29) with the herbal ingredients.

DOSAGE

This formula works best at a higher, more frequent dose. If symptoms are present, be sure to follow the acute dosing guidelines (p. 44).

See Influenza Protocol (p. 86)

IMMUNITY

The Garden of Immuni-Tea

Rustle up some ingredients from your spice cabinet or pick your garden-fresh herbs to concoct this easy-as-can-be brew. Most excellent for when you are feeling the effects of a sore throat, or when a cold is on its way or present. Quite delicious and medicinal – win!

HERBAL INGREDIENTS

2–4 sprigs fresh thyme or 1 teaspoon dried thyme
1 tablespoon fresh oregano or 1 teaspoon dried oregano
3 slices fresh lemon
1–2 teaspoons manuka honey (allow your tea to cool a little before adding, to retain the honey's beneficial enzymes)

METHOD

Make the Medicinal Tea base recipe (p. 33) with the herbal ingredients.

See Acute Colds Protocol (p. 78); Chest Cold Protocol (p. 80)

Garlic in Your Socks

An old folk remedy that keeps on giving! The method is just as simple as the recipe name: pop a few peeled cloves of garlic into a pair of non-precious sleeping socks and let the medicinal magic soak in through the soles of your feet overnight. This uncomplicated act of immune fortification to ward off bugs and viruses is particularly wonderful when a cold or flu is looming or already present.

HERBAL INGREDIENT

2 cloves garlic

METHOD

Before you go to bed, peel the garlic cloves, pop on some socks and position the cloves inside your socks so they are tucked in securely under the arches of your feet. Sleep well!

See Acute Colds Protocol (p. 78)

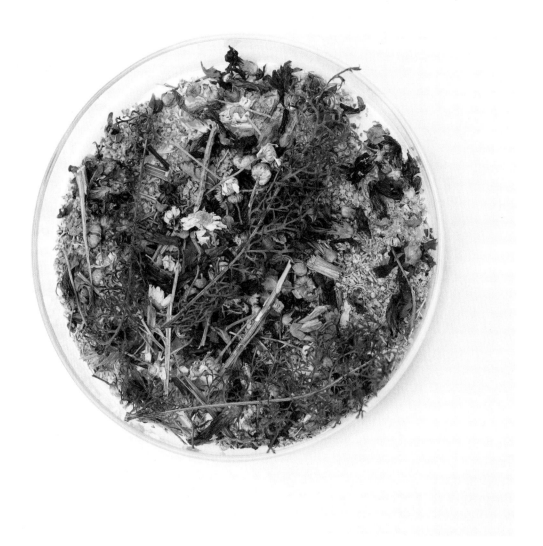

Fever Tea

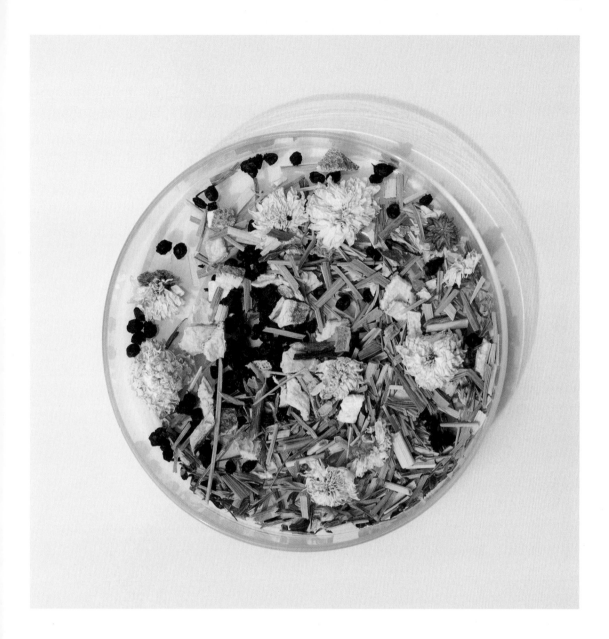

Immune Enhancer Tea

Ginger Bath Bomb

A ginger-imbued bath is a fitting remedy for cold-like symptoms or to pump up detoxification, activating an inner-clearing cascade by increasing the sweat response. Be sure to drink plenty of extra water before, during and after the bath to support your body's lymphatic and cleansing flow.

HERBAL INGREDIENTS

2 tablespoons fresh ginger rhizome or 1–2 teaspoons dried ginger rhizome

½ cup Epsom salts (optional, but will deepen detoxification)

METHOD

Pop the ingredients into a running, hot-as-you-can-handle bath, and soak your body for 20–30 minutes. Soak from the neck down to avoid getting any water in your eyes! This practice is best undertaken in the evening, before getting a good night's rest. Note: It is wise to do a patch test on your arm first, particularly if you have sensitive skin. Just make a quick paste with the ginger and a little water, and apply to your inner arm. Wait a few minutes and wash off. If the skin is irritated, avoid the ginger bath! After your ginger bath, wrap yourself up in warm layers and jump into bed. You may experience continued sweating and an increased sensation of body heat for a few hours – this is completely normal.

See Acute Colds Protocol (p. 78)

Grand Garlic Capsules

Really, we could wax lyrical about garlic's long list of healthful benefits, from its high antioxidant content to the cardiovascular and immune support this gracious bulb offers. Simply put, garlic is a star. This recipe is in capsule form, to help us all bypass the odour challenges that come with eating a tonne of garlic.

HERBAL INGREDIENT

3 tablespoons garlic
   powder

METHOD

Make the Capsules base recipe (p. 29) with the garlic powder.

If you have a dehydrator, peel 20 garlic cloves and dehydrate on the lowest setting to be sure that the garlic retains its medicinal potency. Grind the dried garlic in a clean spice grinder or a mortar and pestle.

If you are purchasing garlic powder, please be sure to choose the best quality possible, as heat treatment will impair some of the medicinal constituents of garlic.

See Chest Cold Protocol (p. 80); Wet Cough Protocol (p. 89)

Guardian Tea

An antiviral powerhouse, blended to create a strong defence in the face of viral presentations, whether that be a cold sore or a viral cold. Licorice, lemon balm, echinacea and St John's wort combine to soothe tension and calm the heightened stress response that often underlies a weakened immune system.

HERBAL INGREDIENTS

1 teaspoon dried St John's
   wort flowers/leaf
1 teaspoon dried
   echinacea leaf/root
½ teaspoon dried
   licorice root
2 teaspoons dried lemon
   balm leaf

METHOD

Make the Medicinal Tea base recipe (p. 33) with the herbal ingredients.

See Cold Sores (p. 122)

Gum to Gut Tea

HERBAL INGREDIENTS

1 teaspoon dried green tea
(omit if you are caffeine-
sensitive, or use rooibos
tea instead)

peel of ½ lemon or citrus
fruit of choice

1 sprig fresh rosemary or
1 teaspoon dried
rosemary

1 cinnamon quill

1 teaspoon dried oregano

1 teaspoon dried thyme

½ small knob fresh ginger
rhizome, sliced or
1 teaspoon dried ginger
rhizome

1 teaspoon dried fennel
seeds

Gum health is intrinsically connected to gut health, and in this tea many of the herbs cross over to impact not only the oral cavity but also the digestive system. Minimising the growth of harmful bacteria is key for oral health! This antioxidant-rich blend is great to make daily, and is full of readily available aromatic kitchen herbs.

METHOD

Make the Decoction base recipe (p. 29) with the herbal ingredients.

See Gingivitis (p. 122)

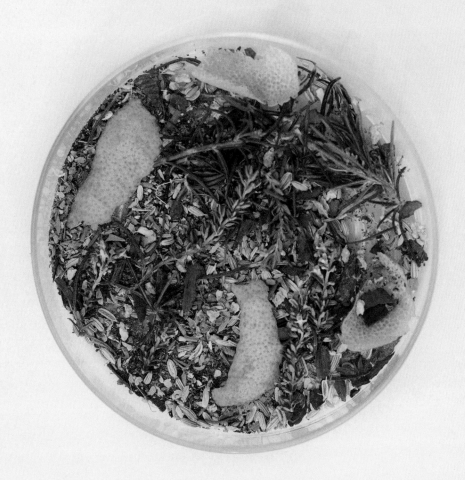

Herbal Fumigation

HERBAL INGREDIENTS

A handful or two of fresh
   or dried rosemary, sage,
   eucalyptus or thyme

Fumigation is the practice of boiling aromatic herbs to clear the air, through the antibacterial action and decongestant properties of the plants. Most fitting when a family member is coming down with a sniffle. Essentially, this is a long-brewed decoction and herbal steam for the home. You can use one herb or a blend.

METHOD

Pop the plant material into a large pot, cover completely with plenty of water and bring to a rapid boil. Allow to boil continuously for 30 minutes to an hour, checking the level of the water in the pan and topping up as needed. The scented steam will permeate the air!

See Influenza Protocol (p. 86)

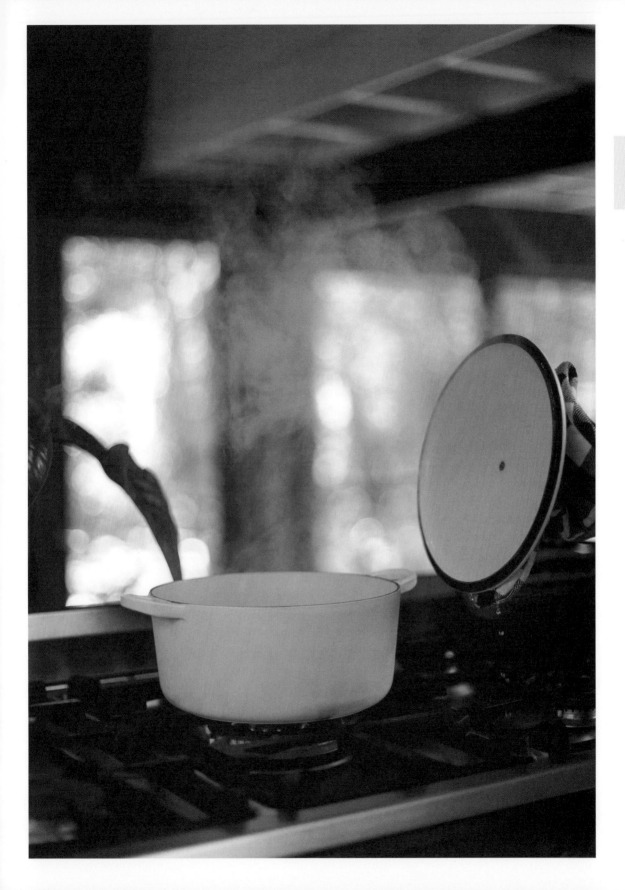

Heroic Herbal Steam Bowl

A great way to ameliorate and clear congestion, the simple act of steaming is an ancient traditional practice in herbalism. This recipe is flexible – you could use fresh or dried herbs, from the garden or the spice cabinet. You can either use one herb, or a combination! Ideal for sinus issues, coughs, colds and flus.

HERBAL INGREDIENTS

¼ cup dried or ½ cup
   fresh aromatic herbs
   (eucalyptus, rosemary,
   thyme, lavender,
   peppermint or oregano
   would be perfect)

METHOD

Place your herbal ingredients in a heatproof bowl, then pour boiling water over the plant material.

A super-important step before putting your precious face anywhere close to the steam is to test the heat by holding your hand over the steamy bowl!

Use a towel to cloak yourself and lean over the bowl, creating a little enclosed steam tent of sorts.

With closed eyes, take deep slow inhalations through the nose for 2–5 minutes. Take a break when needed.

You may find your nasal passages unclog quite promptly!

See Sinus Protocol (p. 88); Wet Cough Protocol (p. 89)

Immune Enhancer Tea

A lively blend for everyday use to upgrade the immune system. With punchy, vitamin C–rich berry and citrus notes, this easy-to-sip tea makes a perfect iced beverage or steamy pot to support you through seasonal changes.

HERBAL INGREDIENTS

1 teaspoon dried
  echinacea root/leaf
1 ½ teaspoons dried
  lemongrass
3 teaspoons dried
  elderberries
1 ½ teaspoons dried
  orange peel
½ teaspoon dried
  chrysanthemum flowers

METHOD

Make the Medicinal Tea base recipe (p. 33) with the herbal ingredients. Be sure to give this blend a solid 20 minutes to steep.

See Influenza Protocol (p. 86)

Lung Love Syrup

When a wet cough is present, this medicinal preparation will combat coughing fatigue and work to get to the roots of any irritation or infection present. With antibacterial and antimicrobial elements, and demulcent and nutrient-dense herbs, this combo is not only therapeutic but also incredibly tasty. Due in part to their treacle-like consistency, which offers welcome relief, syrups are well tolerated when the throat is sore.

HERBAL INGREDIENTS

3 tablespoons dried thyme
3 tablespoons dried
  elderberries
3 tablespoons dried
  rosehips
3 tablespoons dried
  elecampane
4 tablespoons dried
  marshmallow root

METHOD

Make the Simple Syrup base recipe (p. 37) with the herbal ingredients.

See Sinus Protocol (p. 88); Wet cough protocol (p. 89)

Mullein Garlic Ear Oil

For ear aches and pains, drop this simple remedy into the ear canal. Mullein has a true affinity for the ear canal, while garlic works to reduce any potential infection formation and presence. It is best to warm the oil very gently before use. Apply drops frequently when the ear is in need, but please do not use this oil if there is any possibility you might have a perforated eardrum.

HERBAL INGREDIENTS

2 tablespoons dried
   mullein flowers/leaf
2 cloves of peeled and
   sliced garlic

METHOD

Add the herbal ingredients to a double boiler along with 3 tablespoons of olive oil. Simmer over low heat for 15 minutes. Remove from heat and strain through a fine mesh seive. Pour into a sterilsed dropper bottle.

DOSAGE

Lie on your side and drop 3 drops of warm oil into the ear canal. Pop cotton wool into the ear, then maintain your restful horizontal pose for 10 minutes to allow the oil to permeate down the canal. Apply multiple times daily in acute presentations. Also, it is wise to treat both ears!

See Earache (p. 122)

Nasturtium Flower Vinegar

A nasturtium in bloom is a sight to behold! With neon oranges, shocking reds and canary yellows the blooms not only captivate our vision, they also offer us a wealth of medicinal benefits. This simple flower-infused vinegar is beyond pretty – once imbued, the vinegar turns a shade of ruby red. Aesthetics aside, this preparation is a strong antibiotic to fortify immunity and ward off viruses, colds and respiratory infections.

HERBAL INGREDIENT

2 cups fresh nasturtium
   flowers

METHOD

Make the Vinegar base recipe (p. 39) with the nasturtium flowers.

See Sinus Protocol (p. 88); Influenza Protocol (p. 86)

Neti Pot Sinus Rinse

A soothing sinus-specific combination to free up congestion, calm irritation and inflammation, and offer immune-enhancing power to the passages. Such an easy way to encourage the sinuses to drain!

HERBAL INGREDIENTS

2 teaspoons dried olive leaf

2 teaspoons dried mullein leaf

2 teaspoons dried chamomile flowers

2 teaspoons dried ribwort leaf

METHOD

Make the Medicinal Tea base recipe (p. 33) with the herbal ingredients.

Allow the tea to cool and decant into a clean neti pot. Leaning over a basin, tilt your head to the right, position the spout of the neti pot in your right nostril and breathe through your mouth. The plant-infused liquid will irrigate the right nostril and drain out of the left nostril! Repeat on the other side.

DOSAGE

It is best to repeat this rinse at least twice daily when sinuses are impacted.

See Acute Colds Protocol (p. 78); Hay Fever Protocol (p. 85); Sinus Protocol (p. 88)

Nettle, Reishi and Rose Raw Honey

A smooth-tasting trio soaked in the golden nectar of honey. Add to sweeten and nutrify an iced tea or use as a face mask to brighten and nourish the skin. Nettle has a true affinity for allergy and adrenal support, while rose lifts the heart. Drizzle this honey on your morning porridge for a buoyant lift!

HERBAL INGREDIENTS

1 tablespoon nettle leaf powder

1 teaspoon reishi powder

1 ½ tablespoons rose petal powder

METHOD

Make the Electuary base recipe (p. 30) with the herbal ingredients.

See Hay Fever Protocol (p. 85)

Onion and Garlic Honey

A beloved herbalist's trick: we love to douse pungent goods in honey for greater taste compliance! Honey adds its own benefits as it mellows out the flavours of onion and garlic, delivering a smooth spoonful of potent plant medicine. Great for overall immunity, colds, flu, sinus conditions, coughs, raw throats and upper respiratory tract infections.

HERBAL INGREDIENTS

6 cloves garlic, grated
2 brown onions, finely
   sliced

METHOD

Add the garlic and onions to a sterilised jar and top with 1 cup of raw honey and allow to sit at room temperature for 24 hours. This herbal honey is now ready to enjoy. Either strain out the herbal ingredients with a fine-mesh sieve into a fresh sterilised jar or leave them in for an extra bold bite. For longevity store in the fridge for up to 3 months.

See Sinus Protocol (p. 88)

The Orange Orchard Oxymel

With a pop of citrus infused into the golden base of raw honey and apple cider vinegar, this vitamin C–rich blend is the perfect daily medicine to employ over the cooler seasons, lending immune support a mighty hand.

HERBAL INGREDIENTS

3/4 cup dried elderflower
1/4 cup dried orange peel
1 cup dried rosehips
1/2 cup dried echinacea
   root/leaf/flowers

METHOD

Make the Oxymel base recipe (p. 34) with the herbal ingredients.

DOSAGE

Best taken daily when you are seeking immune support. If acute symptoms are present, increase the dose as outlined in the dosing guidelines (p. 45).

See Chronic Low Immunity Protocol (p. 82)

Sage and Saltwater Gargle

Gargling can be a simple frontline intervention when a strained or sore throat is present. You can use many other kitchen herbs in place of sage – try thyme or marjoram if they are on hand.

METHOD

Make the Medicinal Tea base recipe (p. 33) with the herbal ingredients. Allow to cool to a warm temperature and add salt, stirring to combine. Gargle thoroughly – avoid swallowing the liquid. After a thorough swish around the mouth, spit out and repeat.

See Dry Cough Protocol (p. 84)
See also Mouth Ulcers/Canker Sores (p. 123)

HERBAL INGREDIENTS

1 tablespoon dried sage
1 teaspoon salt

Sage Tea

A simple brew with the earthy boldness of sage leaf.

METHOD

Make the Medicinal Tea base recipe (p. 33) with the sage.

See Sore Throat (p. 123)
See also Oversupply of Breast Milk (p. 232)

HERBAL INGREDIENT

2 teaspoons dried sage
or 4 teaspoons fresh sage

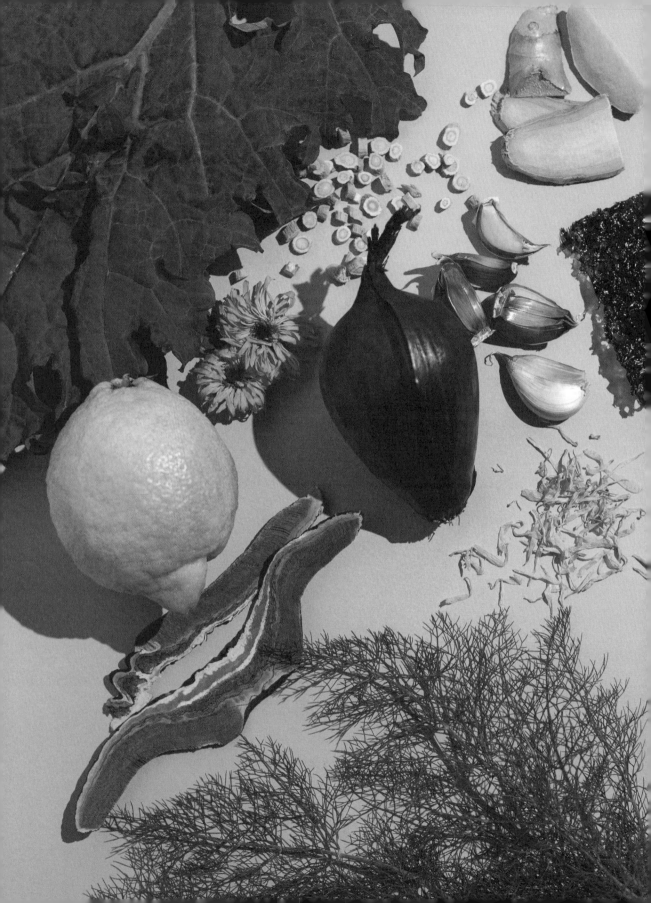

Scrap Broth

A food-waste reduction revelation! Scrap broth is made by combining food scraps with common kitchen ingredients, to yield a nourishing wellspring that can be included on the daily to supercharge nutrition and immunity. This recipe is totally open to interpretation – I strongly encourage you to experiment and to swap out these ingredients for what you may have on hand.

MAKES ABOUT 8 CUPS

HERBAL INGREDIENTS

1–2 tablespoons dried calendula flowers

3 slices dried reishi

1 cup pre-soaked shiitake (soak in hot water for 20 minutes, covered)

2 tablespoons fresh turmeric rhizome, finely chopped, or 1 tablespoon dried turmeric rhizome

1 tablespoon dried astragalus root

1 handful parsley leaf/stem

2 sprigs fresh rosemary or 1 teaspoon dried rosemary

1 small knob fresh ginger rhizome, sliced, or 1 teaspoon dried ginger rhizome

1 whole head garlic, peeled and sliced

2 brown or red onions, sliced or cut into chunks

2 slices dried kombu or a whole wakame sheet, sliced

3 cups fresh or frozen veggie scraps (e.g. broccoli stems, kale ribs and stems, celery tops, sweet potato or carrot peelings, onion skins)

METHOD

Place all the ingredients in a large pot and add 10 cups of water to completely cover. Bring to a full boil, then allow to simmer for 1 hour. If needed, top up with a little more water to ensure the herbal ingredients are well covered.

Remove from the heat. Strain out the herbs and vegetables with a large fine-mesh sieve, allow to cool, then freeze in batches for extended use!

A great way to store your veggie scraps is to seal them in an airtight bag and keep in the freezer.

See Chest Cold Protocol (p. 80); Chronic Low Immunity Protocol (p. 82); Dry Cough Protocol (p. 84); Influenza Protocol (p. 86)
See also Postnatal Depletion Protocol (p. 216); Shingles (p. 268)

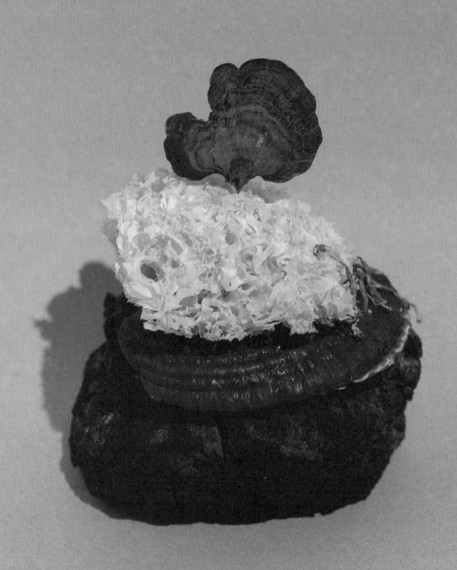

SJW Oil

HERBAL INGREDIENT

2 cups fresh St John's wort
flowers/leaf (you can
use 1 cup dried St John's
wort, but freshly picked is
best in this case)

This is an essential herbal oil to add to your home apothecary!
SJW Oil is imbued with the cheery yellow flowers and feathery
leaves of St John's wort, a common 'weed' that grows
worldwide. The oil turns a deep red once infused. Apply
topically for muscular aches and pains, cold sores, shingles
and neuralgic pain.

METHOD

Make the Herbal-Infused Oil base recipe (p. 31) with the
St John's wort.

See Chickenpox (p. 122); Cold Sores (p. 122)
See also Shingles (p. 268)

Supreme Shrooms

HERBAL INGREDIENTS

½ tablespoon reishi
powder
½ tablespoon maitake
powder
½ tablespoon chaga
powder
½ tablespoon cordyceps
powder
½ tablespoon turkey tail
powder
½ tablespoon lion's mane
powder

An adaptogenic, powdered, encapsulated blend of medicinal
mushrooms to strengthen immunity and fortify longevity. Weave
in to your daily routine to tonify health, or increase to a higher
dose if you're feeling under the weather. It is absolutely fine to
keep this formula in powdered form and add it to a warming
tonic or other drink of choice.

METHOD

Make the Capsules base recipe (p. 29) or the Herbal Powder
base recipe (p. 33) with the herbal ingredients.

See Chronic Low Immunity Protocol (p. 82); Influenza Protocol (p. 86)
See also Longevity Protocol (p. 52)

Rescue Remedies

CHICKENPOX

Often more of an issue for infants and children, chickenpox is caused by the varicella-zoster virus (which is also the cause of shingles). To ease the itching caused by the rash, which can be very uncomfortable and agitating, take a twice-daily **Oaty Bath** (p. 261) – the demulcent goodness of whole oats will soothe irritation and cool the skin. Oil-up the skin with **SJW Oil** (p. 121), which will also promote relaxation for the nervous system. For infants, a cup of **Chamomile Tea** (p. 161) can be very helpful to ease the insidious stress associated with itching. Adults, children and teens can dose up on the **Antiviral Tincture** (p. 246), which promotes prompt movement of the virus (in turn leading to clearance and recovery), as well as immune support and calming of the nervous system. If a fever is present, bring on the **Fever Tea** (p. 102), containing yarrow, elder and peppermint, to assist with fever management.

COLD SORES

Time to bring your antiviral herbs on board with **Guardian Tea** (p. 107), a mix of lemon balm, St John's wort, licorice and echinacea. Sip on this quartet throughout the day. Apply **SJW Oil** (p. 121) topically to your forming or present cold sore, frequently. You could also apply the **Guardian Tea** (p. 107) topically as a wash, to soothe.

PS: Herpes virus is responsible for a cold-sore outbreak. Often this is triggered and exacerbated by stress and exhaustion.

CONJUNCTIVITIS

Brew a strong, warm infusion of **Ease the Eyes Wash** (p. 101) and apply every 2–4 hours if possible. This antimicrobial, soothing combo can work wonders at the onset of infection. Conjunctivitis (also called pinkeye) is highly contagious, so be sure to practise good hygiene.

PS: A little extra liver and immune support is most definitely indicated to shift conjunctivitis.

EARACHE

When an earache looms, it is best to get in swiftly with herbal treatment. Try **Mullein Garlic Ear Oil** (p. 114), an infused oil best dropped into the ear two to three times per day. I suggest warming the oil slightly for a gentle entrance into the ear. This revered folk remedy is perfect for all earache concerns and for warding off infection. Do not apply this treatment if there is any possibility at all that you might have a perforated eardrum.

FEVER

Fever Tea (p. 102), composed of yarrow, elderflower and peppermint, has long been a favourite of herbalists for managing a fever.

GINGIVITIS

The everything-but-the-kitchen-sink **Gum to Gut Tea** (p. 108) is very simple to make. Full of culinary herbs, citrus peel and green tea, this antioxidant, antimicrobial, antibacterial combo aids in the treatment of gingivitis and the maintenance of general oral health.

PS: There is most definitely a positive crossover impact on gut health here. Oral health is deeply interconnected with gut health.

MOUTH ULCERS/CANKER SORES

Use the **Sage and Saltwater Gargle** (p. 117) to rinse your mouth. Rub infused **Clove Oil** (p. 97) directly onto ulcers and sores to soothe as needed throughout your day.

PS: Mouth ulcers and canker sores commonly occur when you are feeling run-down, stressed and weary, and can also be a sign of underlying vitamin deficiencies such as low B12, zinc, iron and folic acid. The hormonal changes preceding a menstrual cycle can sometimes catalyse a mouth ulcer, while underlying food sensitivities are another trigger – if you are frequently experiencing mouth ulcers or canker sores, consider getting your blood work done via your practitioner to check in on optimal levels. Rest, connect with nature to de-stress and tune into self-talk.

SORE THROAT

The simplest intervention for a sore throat is a big teaspoon of high-grade manuka honey – repeat three times daily. Or try **Coat Your Throat Tea** (p. 97), a delicious blend specifically for a sore, irritated throat. I like to rotate the tea with the **Botanical Throat Spray** (p. 91), to really cover all the bases. Or simply make a strong, soothing **Sage Tea** (p. 117).

STAPH INFECTIONS

Complex and tenacious, a staph infection can manifest in many ways, often impacting the skin. Infection caused by staphylococcus bacteria most commonly presents as a minor skin condition, but can certainly escalate to a more serious presentation. Berberine-rich herbs such as goldenseal, or the more sustainable options of barberry or Oregon grape, are key to the treatment of staph infections – alongside garlic and echinacea, which are very helpful here – being used either internally or externally. Tea tree oil and/or eucalyptus oil offer their antibacterial powers when applied topically.

WARTS

Often stubborn and troublesome, warts are caused by the human papillomavirus. This is definitely the time to support immunity, with a daily dose of the **Echinacea Tincture** (p. 101). The most successful topical treatment method known to many herbalists involves good old banana peel. Use the white inner side of a ripe banana peel, taping it onto the wart like a compress. Apply a fresh banana peel daily and persist with this treatment for at least 2–4 weeks, until your wart has cleared.

Detoxification

The good news is that we are innately geared to automate detoxification. Picture the detoxification process being triggered and then working its way through multiple organs and channels to eject toxic substances and metabolites, foreign matter (bacteria, viruses, fungi, cancerous cells and so on) and waste materials. We have multiple ways to excrete toxins and waste via the excretory system, through the liver, the colon, the kidneys, the lungs, the lymphatic system, the blood and the skin. Our breath, sweat, urine and stools are all channels of elimination. We are primed to self-regulate and protect, to constantly aim for homeostasis. So clever!

The not-so-good news is that the body absolutely has its limitations. We are not innately geared to cope with excessive exposure to toxins. This is an especially challenging situation with the world as it is, when so many things affecting our everyday lives – from alcohol to synthetic perfumes to car fumes – create a toxic burden. When our bodies reach the point of needing a helping hand to clear congestion, they will often tell us 'enough is enough'.

Our bodies will speak to us with symptoms. For example, the digestive system may feel somewhat overburdened after a bout of celebratory drinks or a period of eating out of normal range, or the skin may be reactive when the liver is a tad overloaded. These symptoms often represent a clear marker that the body needs extra assistance.

The thing is, there are whole industries built around helping you to detoxify, from 'miracle' weight-loss cures (or so they claim) to stringent liquid-cleanse programs. It can be a confusing minefield to navigate when all you desire is to feel a little clearer in your body and being. In truth, detoxification can be quite simple.

Returning to the Pillars to Thrive (p. 16) is essential. Ensuring that you are drinking enough water and that your bowel elimination is in flow (and not clogged up), as well as eating nutritious foods and moving your body regularly, are incredibly helpful acts of support to kick-start a regenerative cleanse.

Herbal medicine holds a treasure chest of plants that impact the excretory system: plants that speak directly to the liver or engage the lymphatics fluently. So many of these plant medicines are quite common; in fact, some of the best cleansing herbals are deemed 'weeds'. They often magically appear just when needed, popping up in the spring, for example, a time when we wake from a winter slumber with our bodies requiring a little reinvigoration. The synergy of the plants and the people strikes again!

Often all that may be needed to clear the body is to simply unburden the load and work with the plants to amplify a reset.

Consider these easy but effective cleansing tips

— Take your body movement down a notch to a less intensive pace when actively undertaking a detox of any sort. Think walks, yin yoga, swimming, and so on.

— Weave in more relaxation practices, such as breathwork, meditation or qi gong.

— Get into the light of the day. Sunlight not only aids the synthesis of vital vitamin D but also enhances your inner vitality, which is key to supporting a cleanse of any sort. The inherent bonus of this is allowing yourself time in nature to restore and reinvigorate the senses.

— Take stock and edit out anything (within reason for you) that may be burdening you or that you perceive as toxic. This may mean a break from an unhealthy relationship – or simply editing your kitchen cupboards.

— Allow your body and being to rest ... like, really rest! Resting is not just zoning out in front of a screen (although it may look like that for some). You could clear your schedule, read a book outside in the sun, or take a nap.

— Follow the supportive Food is Medicine guidelines (p. 20). Pay extra attention to eating really well – that means high fibre, high hydration and liver-loving cruciferous veggies – and be sure to unburden the liver with an alcohol- and processed food–free period.

— Purchase a tongue scraper. Upon rising (before teeth brushing), scrape away. This is a great way to remove bacteria from the mouth and is an easy extra to add in to support your wellbeing.

Please be mindful

If you are considering a juice or liquid-only cleanse, please be well guided. If you have never done one before, approach it a day at a time rather than embarking on an extensive 5-day (or longer) liquid cleanse. **Scrap Broth** (p. 119) is a nourishing option if you are keen to give your digestive system a little rest. I would also suggest that the cleanse protocols that lie ahead will be most effective if undertaken in tandem with a nourishing diet.

Liver Cleanse

Upon Rising	Morning	
DRINK a tall glass of warm water with 5–10 millilitres (1–2 teaspoons) of unpasteurised raw apple cider vinegar added. If this practice is new to you, start at the lower end of the dosage scale to encourage a gentle acclimatisation of the tastebuds.	**DRINK** the nutrient-dense **Liver-Lovin' Greens Powder** (p. 136). Either combine it with water, alchemising with a vigorous stir, or add it to the **Green Dream Smoothie** (p. 131), to supercharge cleansing actions. **POP** the **Hepato-Cleanse Caps** (p. 134) with a full meal. This antioxidant-laden formula – with globe artichoke, dandelion root, rosemary and schisandra berry – primes liver function and enhances hepatic harmony.	
Enhancements	**CONSIDER** a **Castor Oil Pack** (p. 160), placed on the upper right quadrant of the abdomen, over the liver, to deepen detoxification.	

When the liver is feeling sluggish, it is time for a little extra assistance from the plants. The liver often appreciates a bit of gentle encouragement, to reinforce clearance and reinstate a bright twinkle in the eye. I recommend following this protocol for 7–14 days, but feel free to pick and choose whatever resonates, and go gently.

Throughout the Day	Evening
SIP	**SIP**
a big mug of **Let It Go Tea** (p. 135), fuelled with a fusion of herbs to support and accelerate detoxification. This tea also tastes awesome iced.	**The Golden One** (p. 130), for an evening delight. This turmeric latte is laced with warming spices to shift stagnancy, ward off inflammation and aid liver function.

PRACTISE THE PILLARS

Be sure to meet your daily **HYDRATION** needs to enhance innate detoxification. Eat really nourishing, **GOOD FOOD**. Honour down time and **REST**. Weave in gentle daily **BODY MOVEMENT**. Affirm your liver with positive **SELF-TALK**.

Spring Cleanse

Morning	Throughout the Day
DRINK	**DRESS**
Shifting Stagnancy Tea (p. 141), an awakening blend to cleanse the blood, support the liver and cue vitality. With echinacea, dandelion, cleavers, nettle and more, this earthy blend will clear the cobwebs of seasons past.	your meals and salads with a dash of **Spring Elixir** (p. 143), a vital effervescence captured in an infused apple cider vinegar base. Essentially made with everything that is blooming in the garden, this is spring in a bottle! Infused flowers and leaves imbue the vinegar with life.
	EAT
	wild green weeds and edible flowers. Think dandelion leaf, chickweed, gotu kola, red clover blossoms, calendula petals, nasturtium flowers. As nature wakes up, the plants are ripe with vitality.

Upon spring's arrival, the body beckons us to wake up and shake off the winter slumber. Spring is the perfect time to clear away internal cobwebs and sluggishness. With the land around you mirroring your process, there are plenty of herbs that offer to (quite literally) put the spring back in your step!

Enhancements

PRACTISE THE PILLARS

Keep up **HYDRATION**. Focus on eating nourishing **GOOD FOOD**. Honour down time and **REST**. Weave in daily **BODY MOVEMENT**. Saturate yourself with positive **SELF-TALK**! Be sure to **CONNECT WITH NATURE**, to attune yourself to the awakening and clearing energy of spring.

Deep Forest Tea Blend

HERBAL INGREDIENTS

2 teaspoons dried green
  tea
1 teaspoon dried ginkgo
  leaf
½ teaspoon dried panax
  ginseng root
1 teaspoon dried gotu kola
  leaf
1 ½ teaspoons dried
  rosehips

Antioxidants are essential allies in our quest for longevity and offer a lovely load of reparative elements. Many of the plants in this blend have promising radioprotective properties that work to counteract the effects of exposure to radiation and EMFs (electric and magnetic fields), so you could employ this super-green blend to balance screen fatigue and inject a little energy buzz into your day. Be mindful that green tea does contain caffeine, and ginseng certainly elevates innate energy, so keep this blend for early in your day.

METHOD

Make the Medicinal Tea base recipe (p. 33) with the herbal ingredients.

See Screen Exposure (p. 144)

The Golden One

HERBAL INGREDIENTS

½ teaspoon turmeric
  powder
¼ teaspoon ginger powder
¼ teaspoon cinnamon
  powder
¼ teaspoon cardamom
  powder
a pinch of ground black
  pepper
a dash of raw honey or
  sweetener of choice

Elevate internal warmth and awaken slumbering vibrancy with this sunshine-embodying anti-inflammatory turmeric tonic. A perfect cosy beverage for cool weather – or for those with cooler constitutions. Turmeric loves to be paired with beneficial fats and black pepper to enhance bioavailability. Use a rich coconut milk as the base or add a dash of ghee to activate the golden root.

METHOD

Make the Plant Mylk Tonic base recipe (p. 35) with the herbal ingredients.

See Liver Cleanse Protocol (p. 126)
See also Endurance Support (p. 74)

Green Dream Smoothie

Super green, fibre-dense and grounding – and super versatile. You can substitute your frozen fruit of choice, be that banana, mango or berries, or opt for a low-fructose option such as avocado. You can even add in different veggies, cucumber or fresh mint.

MAKES 1 SERVE

NUTRITIONAL INGREDIENTS

1 teaspoon chlorophyll
  liquid (optional, lends a
  minty flavour)
1 teaspoon chia seeds
1 teaspoon chlorella
  powder or any super-
  greens powder of choice
2 heaped tablespoons
  hemp protein powder
¼ cup shredded coconut
1 cup organic spinach or
  frozen spinach
1–2 frozen bananas
2 cups filtered water or
  plant mylk

METHOD

Simply place the ingredients in a blender and blend on high until smooth.

See Liver Cleanse Protocol (p. 126)
See also Dull Skin Protocol (p. 238)

A little tip: Chew your smoothie to aid digestion.

DETOXIFICATION

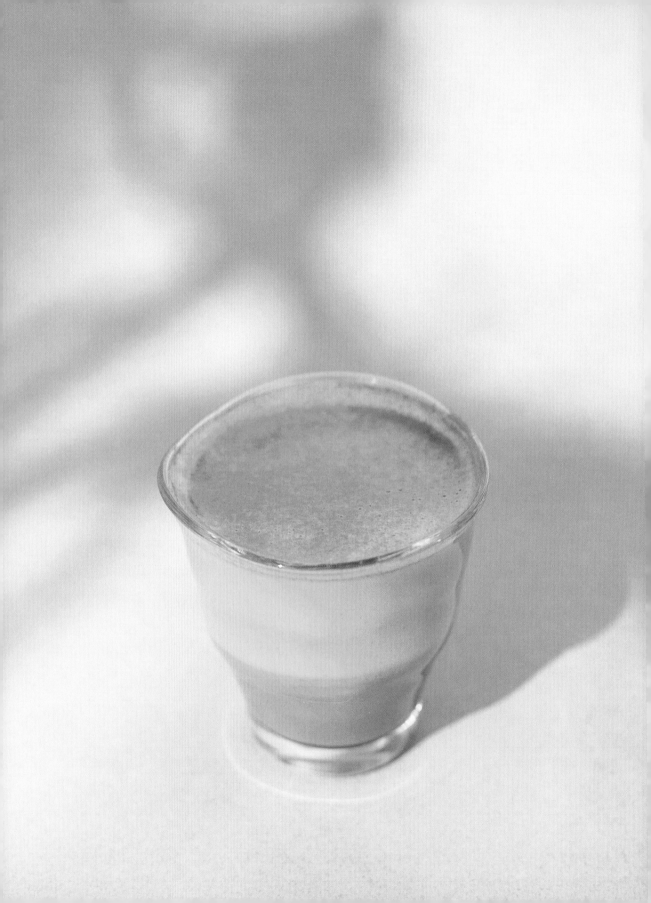

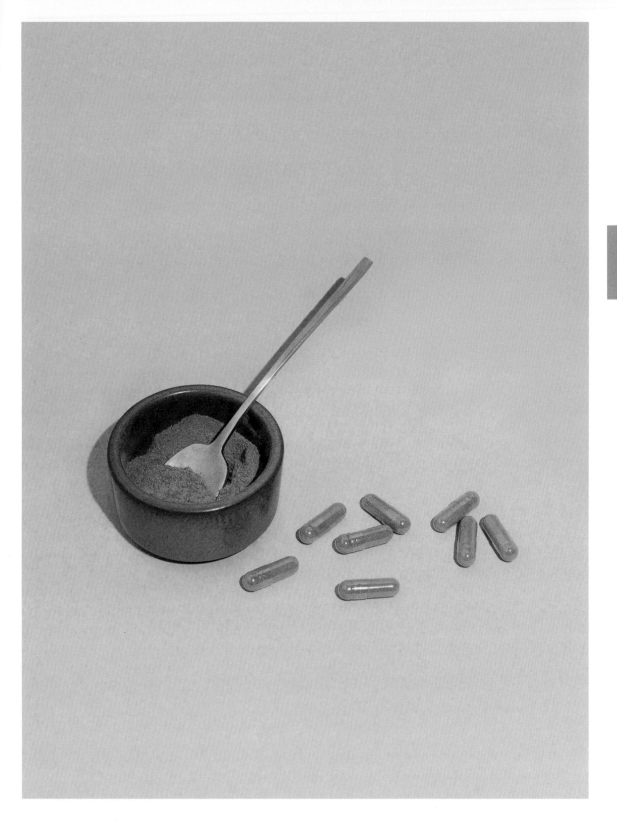

ABOVE *Hepato-Cleanse Caps*

OPPOSITE *The Golden One*

Hepato-Cleanse Caps

HERBAL INGREDIENTS

1 tablespoon dandelion
   root powder
½ tablespoon globe
   artichoke powder
1 tablespoon schisandra
   berry powder
½ tablespoon rosemary
   powder

This is a solid herbal formula to support that masterful metaboliser and detoxifier – the liver! Capsules allow this rather intense flavour combination to smoothly bypass your tastebuds. Rosemary brings her antioxidant-rich, tonifying support; globe artichoke pumps up bile flow; dandelion root strengthens the hepatobiliary system (the liver, gall bladder and bile ducts); and schisandra berry enlivens the liver.

METHOD

Make the Capsules base recipe (p. 29) with the herbal ingredients.

DOSAGE

If you are actively working on enhancing liver clearance and aiding pathways of detoxification, be sure to be consistent with this formula and work with the higher acute-dosing guidelines (p. 44). However, it is always wise to start at a lower dose when working on the liver, and then build up the dose gently.

See Liver Cleanse Protocol (p. 126)
See also Acne Protocol (p. 236)

Let It Go Tea

HERBAL INGREDIENTS

1 teaspoon dried St Mary's
thistle seeds

2 teaspoons dried ginger
rhizome

2 teaspoons rooibos

½ teaspoon ground black
pepper

1 teaspoon dried
schisandra berries

1 teaspoon dried goji
berries

1 teaspoon dried burdock
root

2 teaspoons dried star
anise

A spicy, warming ignition, this beloved blend awakens the liver and innate detoxification. Full of movement catalysers, it is the antidote to stagnancy, helping the body to release and clear. With key liver-loving herbs – St Mary's thistle seed, schisandra berry, ginger and burdock root – this blend is balanced with a chai-like flavoured twist. So good – hot, cool or iced.

METHOD

Make the Decoction base recipe (p. 29) with the herbal ingredients.

See Liver Cleanse Protocol (p. 126)

DETOXIFICATION

Liver-Lovin' Greens Powder

Enhance innate detoxification with this easy-to-concoct plant powder. Weave it into your daily rhythms to unburden sluggishness, add verdant nutrition and bring gentle clearance. There are many complex and costly detox powders on the market these days, but in truth you can alchemise and DIY this recipe with ease. Wonderful added in to boost a smoothie or juice, this nutrient-dense blend offers an overall cleansing impact on the body, supporting the liver and overall digestion while adding antioxidants, and multiple essential minerals and vitamins.

HERBAL INGREDIENTS

1 tablespoon spinach
   powder
2 tablespoons broccoli
   powder
2 tablespoons alfalfa
   powder
2 tablespoons burdock
   root powder
1 tablespoon peppermint
   powder
2 tablespoons papaya leaf
   powder
2 tablespoons nettle
   powder
fruit powders or a pinch
   of stevia leaf powder to
   sweeten (optional)

METHOD

Make the Herbal Powder base recipe (p. 33) with the herbal ingredients.

See Liver Cleanse Protocol (p. 126)
See also Psoriasis Protocol (p. 242)

Note: *If you are sensitive to oxalates, please be mindful that this blend is oxalate-rich.*

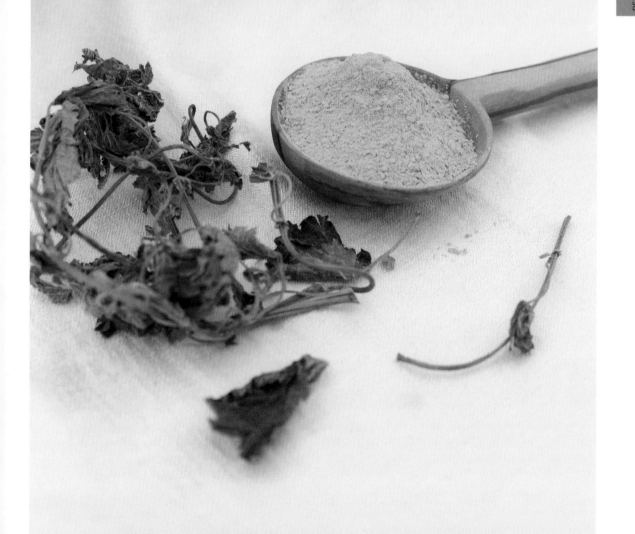

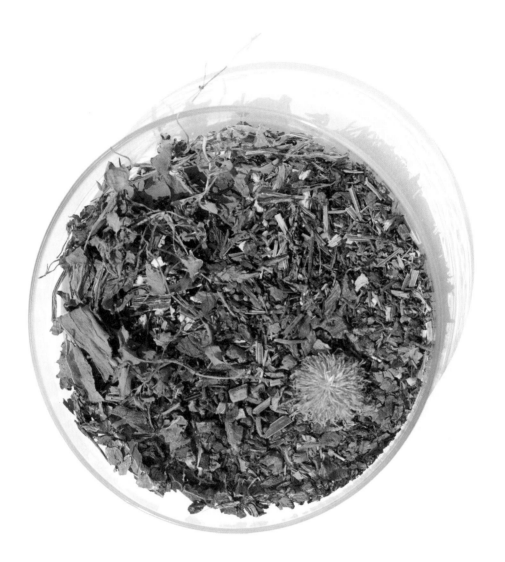

Shifting Stagnancy Tea

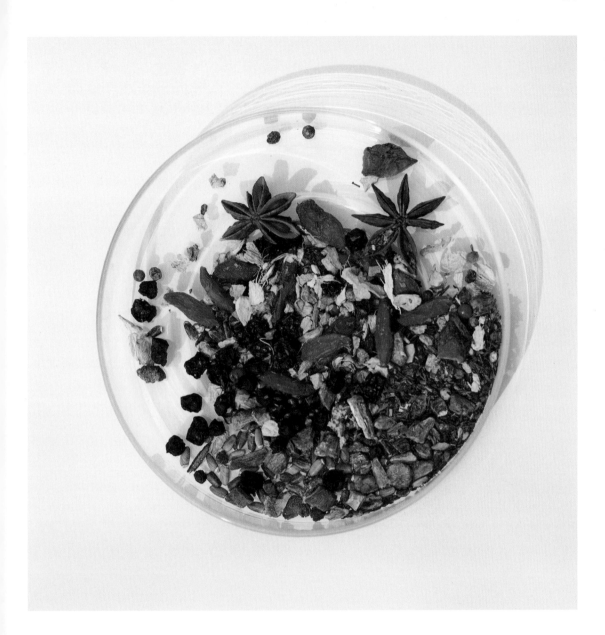

Let It Go Tea

Lung Purifier Syrup

HERBAL INGREDIENTS

4 tablespoons dried
   mullein leaf
4 tablespoons dried
   marshmallow root
2 tablespoons dried thyme
2 tablespoons dried
   hibiscus flowers
4 tablespoons dried linden
   flowers
3 tablespoons dried
   aniseed
2 tablespoons dried
   St Mary's thistle seeds

An entirely nourishing and moistening remedy for the throat and lungs. Utilise this blend after environmental exposure to smoke, toxins or conditions that may impart dryness to the passages. Reishi mushroom and linden flower offer an underlying network of soft support to calm stress and tension; thyme comes in with her immune support; milk thistle helps in cleansing the liver; and mullein, marshmallow and aniseed soothe lung tissues to promote easeful breath.

METHOD

Make the Simple Syrup base recipe (p. 37) with the herbal ingredients.

See Smoke and Pollution Exposure (p. 144)

Shifting Stagnancy Tea

A superb lymphatic blend, to cleanse the blood and assist with sluggishness. This is a most fitting blend to welcome in a deeper layer of clearing and cleansing for the body – add in seasonally to clear the internal cobwebs. Blood-cleansing herbs are generally wonderful for skin conditions, encouraging tissue-cleansing mechanisms via the lymphatic system.

HERBAL INGREDIENTS

2 teaspoons dried
    echinacea root/leaf
1 teaspoon dried cleavers
    stem/leaf/seeds
2 teaspoons dried
    dandelion leaf/flowers
½ teaspoon dried yellow
    dock root
1 teaspoon dried
    chickweed (fresh is extra
    wonderful if accessible)
3 teaspoons dried nettle
    leaf

METHOD

Make the Medicinal Tea base recipe (p. 33) with the herbal ingredients.

See Spring Cleanse Protocol (p. 128)
See also Dull Skin Protocol (p. 238)

DETOXIFICATION

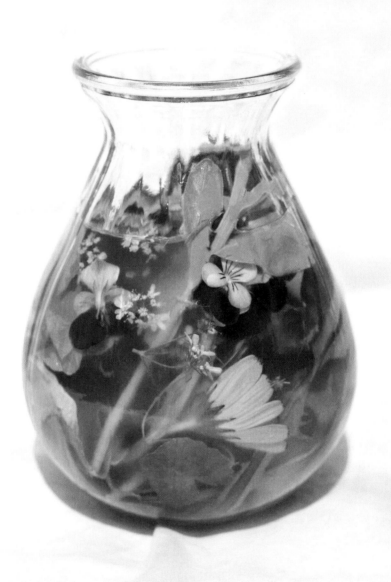

Spring Elixir

Springtime brings a glorious awakening after the slumber of winter. Flowers find their buds and a choir of colours emerge. This recipe concept is an invitation to pick whatever is in bloom and bountiful, essentially submerging your medicinal plant material in apple cider vinegar to infuse the sustenance of spring in a bottle. Be aware – it is essential to identify all your harvested plants with care and certainty, to be sure that they are edible and safe!

This is not so much a structured recipe, more of a really wonderful exercise in connection, communion and appreciation for the plant world. Wherever you may be planted, there will be abundant plant life around you – whether that is to be found in your garden or on a neighbourhood walk. Nasturtiums, dandelion leaves, nettles, cleavers, violets, calendula, elderflower and so much more are all nourishing springtime features to infuse, making a beautiful wild arrangement of medicinal benefits. Reach for your springtime elixir when you need to harness the essence of emergence.

METHOD

Fill a mason jar three-quarters full with fresh plant material and follow the Vinegar base recipe (p. 39).

See Spring Cleanse Protocol (p. 128)

DETOXIFICATION

Rescue Remedies

SCREEN EXPOSURE

Many of us spend the bulk of our days working on screens. Welcome in the **Deep Forest Tea Blend** (p. 130), an antioxidant-rich concoction to protect cellular health and defend you against screen fatigue. With green tea, ginkgo, ginseng and rosehips, this zesty blend also elevates vitality and brings a little pep to your step. Be sure to regularly combat the ill effects of screen time by connecting to nature – get outside, inhale the scents of a blooming flower, kick your shoes off and breathe deeply to regenerate and reset.

SMOKE AND POLLUTION EXPOSURE

Keep the **Lung Purifier Syrup** (p. 140) on hand. With moistening mullein, marshmallow, hibiscus, linden and more, this syrup offers a supportive chalice when needed.

Connecting to *breath*

No matter where you may be, whether that place is quiet or chaotic, the simplest way to calm your body is by connecting with your breath.

Close your eyes and direct your attention inwards. Take a slow deep breath in through the nose, bring it down through the belly, then allow your breath to fill the chest and travel upwards and out through the mouth. Stay with the breath and cycle through until you feel a sense of calm.

You are now connected.

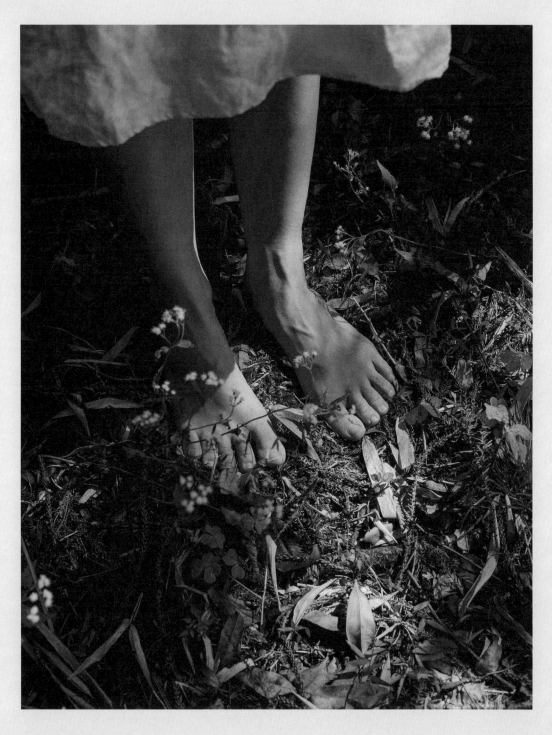

Get out into nature

The Gut

There are many things that can go awry in this delicate area of the body. I find this is more often the case with very sensitive people. The gut is very closely linked to our emotional wellbeing, and if you are a 'feeler' you often may 'feel it' in this tender spot.

The process of digestion involves more than just the stomach, small intestine and large intestine. Yes, it does require a collective effort from these organs – but the pharynx, the oesophagus and the digestive system's accessory organs (the salivary glands, pancreas, liver and gall bladder) are also implicated. The mighty gut – such a remarkable embodiment of organ and system connectivity!

Think of your gut as being foundational, much like a tree's root system, which must remain strong and fortified in order for all other parts – the trunk, the branches, the leaves, the fruit, the flowers – to thrive. In the same way, it is essential to tend to your gut, which impacts all the other areas of your body and being (often in a negative way, when it is off-kilter).

The six Pillars to Thrive (p. 16) are all key practices to bring on board for a healthy gut. Exposure to more natural environmental diversity – simply put, spending more time in nature – plays an important part in animating a healthy microbiome, as does eating foods that heal the gut and keeping yourself hydrated. Even better, time spent in nature helps to reduce stress levels – as the gut/brain axis is majorly influenced by all things stress-related, this is a huge extra benefit!

In this section I have covered many of the most common health imbalances within the digestive system, the spectrum ranging from a slower bowel (constipation) to bad breath (which is most definitely linked to digestive health). It's worth noting that if you are experiencing chronic symptoms, you might want to consider potential underlying digestive dysbioses, such as leaky gut syndrome; food intolerances; yeast, bacterial or parasitic overgrowth; or small intestinal bacterial overgrowth (SIBO). Please see a rad herbalist, naturopath or holistic medicine practitioner to seek diagnosis and clarity if you're worried you have any of these.

Be aware that your stools can tell you a lot about your health. Although this concept may gross you out, it is actually a wise thing to pay attention to them when you go to the loo. Check out the Bristol stool chart (a very helpful clinical tool, beloved by practitioners) to quickly assess whether your stools are healthful – or whether extra care and attention is required to recalibrate your bowels.

So ... into the gut we go!

Consider these actions when you are experiencing digestive symptoms aplenty

— Take a closer look at your diet and see if you notice symptoms that might indicate sensitivity to certain foods; if so, remove and reduce. A great place to start is stripping back known gut irritants (see p. 21).

— Focus on eating slow-cooked, warming foods, such as soups, stews, curries and broths, which are easy to digest. They offer a gallery of other benefits, ranging from support for your gut, immune and adrenal systems to a grounding effect on your nervous system. For a quick, low-fuss option, cook the soups, stews etc. in advance and freeze them in easily accessible meal-size portions.

— Supercharge your nutritional supplementation to support gut health. Glutamine, zinc, vitamin A and omega-3 fatty acids – to name just a few – all have an affinity for healing the gut.

Bloating

Before Each Meal	Morning	
DOSE UP on a shot of **Spiced Herbal Bitters** (p. 171), to awaken digestive power. Take a dose 15–30 minutes before each meal to enhance the production of digestive juices and the breakdown of food.	**DRINK** warm water with a squeeze of lemon juice or 5–10 millilitres (1–2 teaspoons) of unpasteurised raw apple cider vinegar upon rising. **BLEND** yourself a **Gut-Healing Smoothie** (p. 168) for a morning digestive delight. The powerful pairing of calming chamomile and anti-inflammatory turmeric assists with deep repair and digestion. You could also add a serve of **Gut-Healing Powder** (p. 165) to your smoothie.	
Enhancements	**EAT** cooked, warming, nourishing food as the focus of the bulk of your meals – they are super-easily digested when your belly is feeling burdened. Be mindful of avoiding complex food combinations.	

When the belly is feeling burdened and sluggish, and bloating is a frequent visitor, bring these medicinal plant concoctions on board to support and alleviate.

Throughout the Day	Evening
SIP a strongly brewed pot of **CCF Tea** (p. 161), to rebuild digestive fire.	**SIP** a cup of **Bloat-Ease Tea** (p. 156), to relieve any end-of-day bloating and encourage happy dinner digestion.

PRACTISE THE PILLARS

Focus on **HYDRATING** aplenty. **REST** and digest: sit while you eat. When eating, chew thoroughly – and avoid any screens, work or stressful conversations and thoughts.

DAILY PROTOCOL

Constipation

Morning	Throughout the Day	
DRINK upon rising warm water with a squeeze of lemon juice or 5–10 millilitres (1–2 teaspoons) of unpasteurised raw apple cider vinegar. **SIP** a big glass of **Bubble Iced Tea** (p. 158). When soaked in a liquid, chia morphs from solid, hard seeds into soft, hydrophilic (water-absorbent), jelly-like 'bubbles', which add absorbable bulk and fibre as they transit through the digestive system.	**DRINK** a pot of strong **Bloat-Ease Tea** (p. 156), to relieve any feelings of tummy congestion.	
Enhancements	**EAT** an increased amount of fibre-rich foods, to support bowel flow. These come in the form of veggies, fruits, nuts, seeds and whole grains. Add in prebiotic- and probiotic-rich foods (see p. 20).	

A bunged-up belly can plague your day. If this is a chronic issue, it can be the source of frustration and angst. Ideally, we need to move our bowels every day, from one to three times daily. It is so important to unplug stagnation of the bowel – once your bowels recalibrate, you will have renewed pep in your step and experience a sense of lightness. The troublesome stasis can often be caused by the simplest things, such as dehydration or a lack of dietary fibre.

	Afternoon	Evening
	EAT	**PACK**
	Fibre-Dense Bars (p. 164), to increase your intake of dietary fibre. Full of stool-softening elements, these bars will assist a smoother, more easeful elimination process.	a **Castor Oil Pack** (p. 160) on your abdomen if things are extra dire on the no-movement front. An ancient practice among many cultures, the application of packs aids the rhythmic movement of the smooth muscle tissue in the gut (a process known as peristalsis), to support evacuation of the bowels. Once your bowels normalise, you will forget about the oily mess the pack creates.

THE GUT

PRACTISE THE PILLARS

HYDRATION aplenty is an essential remedy for constipation. **REST** and digest. Eat at the same time every day to give the bowel a schedule. Reduce stress and tension with **BODY MOVEMENT** and by stepping outside to **CONNECT WITH NATURE.**

Diarrhoea

Morning and Evening	Throughout the Day
DRINK a tall glass of **Gut-Healing Powder** (p. 165) mixed in water – be sure to have it straight away. The calming and demulcent nature of aloe vera, slippery elm and marshmallow powders speaks to the belly gently yet proficiently. **EAT** super-simple foods, and remove refined and known gut-irritating foods (see p. 21) from your diet. 'Neutral' foods, such as a bowl of white rice, can be comforting for an acute reactive belly.	**DRINK** a few cups of strongly brewed **Astringent Belly Tea** (p. 156). Its astringent properties help to efficiently calm acute diarrhoea. **EAT** grated apple. Leave the grated apple for an hour or so to oxidise and turn a little brown, then add a dash of honey on top – and eat. Sounds a tad unappetising, but it will bind stool very efficiently.

A dodgy belly can stop your day in its tracks. There really is nothing worse than having your confidence in going out in public stymied by your need to know where the nearest bathroom is, at any given moment! Loose stools can be a frequent presentation for many people. Although diarrhoea often hints at a deeper level of health imbalance, you can experience an acute onset as a result of dietary changes, a belly bug, stress or heightened emotions.

Enhancements

PRACTISE THE PILLARS

Focus on **HYDRATION**. It is incredibly important to avoid dehydration, particularly during acute diarrhoea episodes, so drink fluids aplenty. **REST** up to avoid depletion. Stress can often be a big trigger for diarrhoea. Do your best to monitor and ease stress levels where possible.

Indigestion

Acid reflux and persistent heartburn are usually associated with a sensation of acidity and burning that radiates through the chest, which can be incredibly uncomfortable. Indigestion often stems from nutritional choices and a stressed body and being. Making poignant changes to your nutrition and lifestyle, and bringing the herbals on board, can provide a powerful positive shift in your digestive health.

Before Each Meal	Throughout the Day
DOSE UP on the **Botanical Bitters** (p. 157), mixed in a dash of warm water. Take the bitters 15–30 minutes before main meals, to correct digestion. If this worsens the sensation of acidity, please avoid using this remedy.	**DRINK** several cups of soothing **Chamomile Tea** (p. 161), to settle the belly. **POP** the **Neutraliser Capsules** (p. 170). Take with your meals, to soothe and to assist with breakdown of foods and ease of digestion.

Enhancements

PRACTISE THE PILLARS

Breathe deeply before each meal. **REST** when digesting: sit, chew, remove stressors around mealtimes and never eat on the run! Practise mindfulness and **CONNECT WITH NATURE** daily, for a reprieve that will dissipate gut-bothering stress.

EAT

an anti-inflammatory diet that is rich in wholefoods, beneficial fats, quality proteins, and the entire rainbow of low-acid fruits and green veggies. Remove acid-forming provokers such as processed foods, caffeine, alcohol, dairy, gluten and sugars. Be sure to stay hydrated, but avoid drinking liquids with your food, as this can water-down digestive power.

DAILY PROTOCOL

Nausea

Nausea is experienced for many different reasons, ranging from simply eating an overly rich meal to having underlying appetite irregularities (such as those associated with digestive issues, depression and certain emotional states). Or it might occur because you are pregnant and experiencing morning sickness; if so, see the 'Mums and Bubs' section for pregnancy-friendly support. Carminative herbs are the stars here, easing waves of nausea and centring and calming the belly.

Morning, Afternoon and Evening	Throughout the Day
SPOON the **Mint Julep Oxymel** (p. 170), a peppermint- and spearmint-infused burst of goodness that calms queasiness.	**DRINK** fresh **Ginger Tea** (p. 165), an effective reliever to dissipate the waves of nausea.

Enhancements

PRACTISE THE PILLARS

Stay very **HYDRATED,** sipping on water throughout your day – dehydration can cause nausea and increase its severity. Eat **GOOD FOOD,** sticking to smaller, more frequent meals and leaning on the blander side of food choices to calm an unsettled gut.

CONSIDER

acupuncture points to relieve nausea.

Astringent Belly Tea

For when the belly is burdened with the runs, or looser stools are present and persistent. This blend has a super-helpful astringent impact on the gut.

HERBAL INGREDIENTS

1 tablespoon dried
 raspberry leaf
1 tablespoon dried
 blackberry leaf

Note: If you prefer, you can just go with a single herb.

METHOD

Make the Medicinal Tea base recipe (p. 33) with the herbal ingredients.

DOSAGE

Drink ½–1 cup hourly until acute symptoms ease.

See Diarrhoea Protocol (p. 152)

Bloat-Ease Tea

For the distended, sluggish belly. This carminative-rich combination not only tastes delicious, but also aids digestion and reduces acute bloating. A lovely after-dinner blend!

HERBAL INGREDIENTS

1 teaspoon dried
 chamomile flowers
½ teaspoon dried
 meadowsweet flowers/
 leaf
½ teaspoon dried fennel
 seeds
¼ teaspoon dried ginger
 rhizome
½ teaspoon dried
 spearmint leaf
½ teaspoon dried
 peppermint leaf

METHOD

Make the Medicinal Tea base recipe (p. 33) with the herbal ingredients.

DOSAGE

Drink 1 cup after each meal, or whenever you may be feeling digestively challenged.

See Bloating Protocol (p. 148); Constipation Protocol (p. 150)

Botanical Bitters

Our modern diets often lack bitterness. Arouse digestion in the most profound way with this broad-spectrum aperitif. Aimed at encouraging assimilation of nutrients with a botanical bang of bitter flavour, this is perfect for a sluggish digestive system.

HERBAL INGREDIENTS

½ cup dried fennel seeds
½ cup dried chamomile flowers
½ cup dried peppermint leaf
½ cup dried mugwort leaf

METHOD

Make the Tincture base recipe (p. 38) with the herbal ingredients.

DOSAGE

1 teaspoon best taken 15–30 minutes before a meal or as needed, a maximum of three times daily.

See Indigestion Protocol (p. 154)
See also Low Appetite (p. 172)

THE GUT

Bubble Iced Tea

Soaked chia seeds add extra fibre and encourage easy transit of stools, helping to overcome constipation with their mucilaginous goodness. This refreshing herbal-tea base pairs particularly well with chia seeds. You can add chia seeds to any cooled herbal infusion, creating an instant bubble tea.

HERBAL INGREDIENTS

1 tablespoon pineapple chips

1 tablespoon mallow flowers

3 tablespoons ginger rhizome

1 tablespoon linden flowers

2 heaped teaspoons chia seeds

METHOD

Make the Medicinal Tea base recipe (p. 33) with the herbal ingredients to make the tea base.

Allow the tea to cool completely, then strain out the herbs with a fine-mesh sieve.

Add chia seeds to a clean jar or bottle, then pour the strained and cooled tea over.

Give the mixture a little stir, and seal with lid.

Pop in the fridge for at least 4 hours or overnight, to allow the chia seeds to fully soak and soften.

Shake the iced tea, and then sip mindfully. Drinking this through an eco straw feels extra fun!

DOSAGE

Drink 1–3 cups daily, to add fibre and encourage bowel flow.

See Constipation Protocol (p. 150)

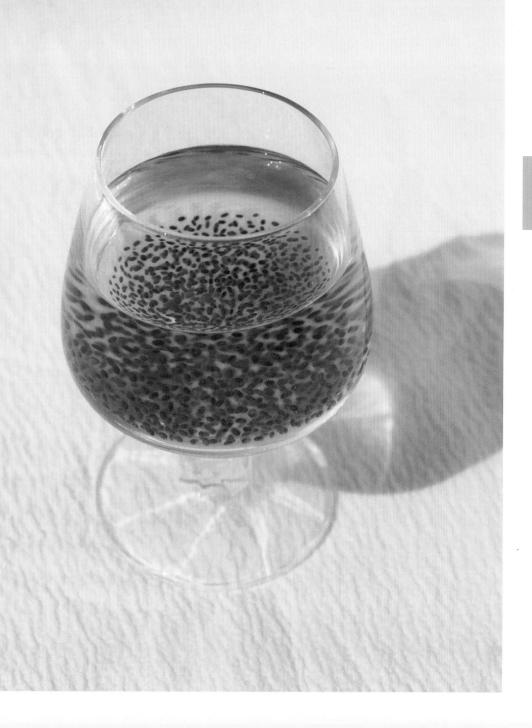

Castor Oil Pack

INGREDIENTS

small bowl of castor oil

EQUIPMENT

hot-water bottle or heat
  pack
old clothes and an old
  towel
a plastic bag or plastic
  wrap

*Cautionary note: In
certain circumstances, it is
recommended that you do not
use castor oil packs. Please
avoid using them if you have an
IUD, or if you are menstruating,
pregnant, lactating or have
an underlying irritable bowel
disorder such as ulcerative
colitis or Crohn's disease.*

Messy but effective, castor oil packs have been utilised over the ages for constipation relief and liver cleansing, tissue and adhesion healing, and enhanced blood flow and circulation, as well as the treatment of joint pain, and menstrual-cycle imbalances such as endometriosis and uterine fibroids. If chronic constipation is a concern, give this a go.

METHOD

Prep your hot-water bottle or heat pack.

Get into your old comfy clothes and prep your space by laying your old towel down. You want to choose a cosy place to do this but one where you can easily wipe down any castor oil spillage. Alternatively, cover the surface with ample old towels to prevent any oil stains!

Bring all of the elements within reach: the castor oil, your heat pack or hot-water bottle, and your plastic bag or plastic wrap.

Lie down on your back, ensuring the towel is positioned across your lower- to mid-back region.

Rub castor oil directly onto the area of your body in need (for constipation, rub directly on the belly) and top with the plastic bag or plastic wrap. Wrap the old towel around your midsection to cover the area being treated, then add the hot-water bottle/heat pack on top.

Leave this on for 30–60 minutes, then dismantle the castor oil pack and wipe any residual oil from your body.

Repeat daily for 1–2 weeks until symptoms improve.

See Constipation Protocol (p. 150)

CCF Tea

An Ayurvedic treasure, this culinary spice combo restores and rebuilds inner digestive power. Consider this blend a reanimator of the digestive system.

HERBAL INGREDIENTS

1 teaspoon coriander
  seeds
1 teaspoon cumin seeds
1 teaspoon fennel seeds

METHOD

Make the Decoction base recipe (p. 29) with the herbal ingredients.

DOSAGE

Drink up to 3 full cups throughout your day.

See Bloating Protocol (p. 148)

Chamomile Tea

A classic! This simple chamomile tea is the most excellent easer of a nervous belly or held tension. Brew well and bliss out.

METHOD

Make the Medicinal Tea base recipe (p. 33) with the chamomile flowers.

HERBAL INGREDIENT

2 heaped teaspoons
  chamomile flowers

DOSAGE

Drink 1–4 cups daily.

See Indigestion Protocol (p. 154)
See also Burnout Protocol (p. 48); Chickenpox (p. 122); Teething (p. 233)

THE GUT

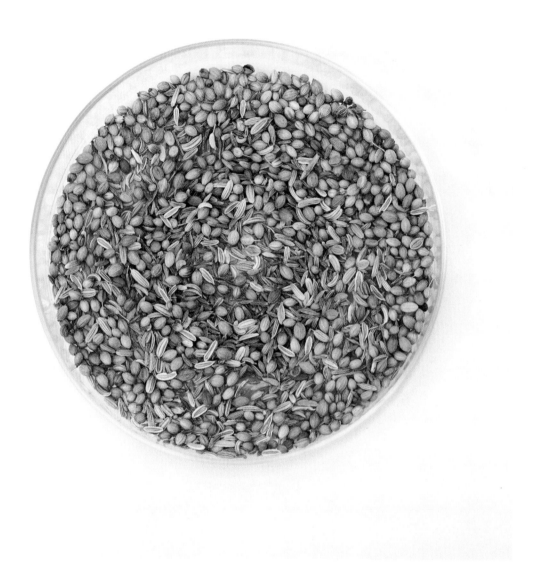

CCF Tea

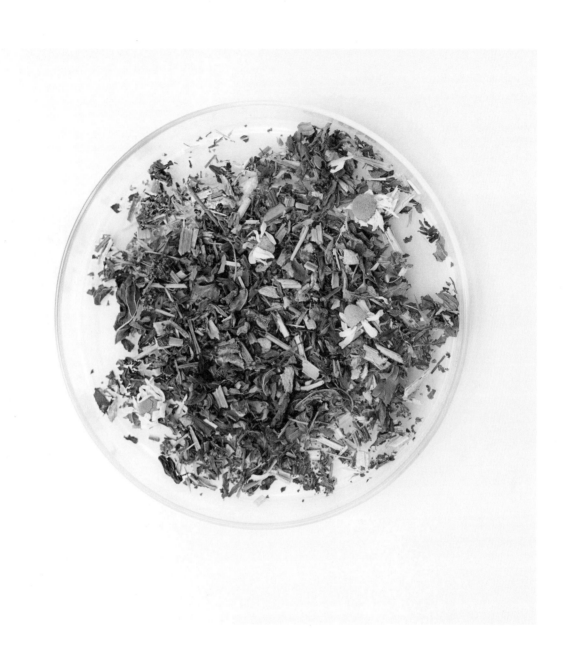

Bloat-Ease Tea

Fibre-Dense Bars

HERBAL INGREDIENTS

1 tablespoon ginger
   rhizome powder
½ tablespoon clove
   powder

NUTRITIONAL INGREDIENTS

1 cup pitted prunes
6 dried figs, roughly
   chopped
1½ cups whole rolled
   gluten-free oats
2 tablespoons almond
   butter
3 tablespoons chia seeds
3 tablespoons psyllium
   powder
½ cup flax seeds
¼ cup melted coconut oil
¼ cup raw honey
a pinch of salt

This raw fruit–laden bar offers a solid dose of dietary fibre and natural bowel-bulking elements to encourage healthy stools, with added ginger and clove to warm the belly. Perfect to bring on board when constipation is present.

MAKES APPROXIMATELY 8 BARS

METHOD

Mash the prunes in a large bowl.

Add the rest of the ingredients to the mashed prune mixture and combine thoroughly.

Spoon into a 20 x 20 centimetre (8 x 8 inch) brownie pan lined with baking paper. Smooth the top of the mixture by gently pressing with the base of a large metal spoon.

Pop in the fridge and allow to chill for 2 hours, or until completely firm.

Slice into squares. Store in a sealed container in the fridge for 1 week, or keep in the freezer and defrost squares for 10 minutes as needed.

DOSAGE

Enjoy 1–3 bars daily!

See Constipation Protocol (p. 150)

Ginger Tea

A no-fuss kitchen-ingredient remedy holding a force-field of healing within, ginger is readily accessible and quick to prepare as a tea. Most wonderful for digestive complaints, from nausea to motion and morning sickness, and to ease flatulence. Also ideal for when a cold looms.

HERBAL INGREDIENT

1 small knob fresh ginger
   rhizome, sliced, or
   1 tablespoon dried
   ginger rhizome

METHOD

Make the Decoction base recipe (p. 29) with the ginger rhizome.

DOSAGE

Enjoy 1–3 cups daily.

See Nausea Protocol (p. 155)
See also Fortified Pregnancy Support Protocol – For Morning Sickness (p. 212); Vomiting (p. 172)

Gut-Healing Powder

A demulcent herbal trio to coat the gastrointestinal system. Perfect for healing the gut and aiding bowel-flow harmony, while soothing digestive issues such as reflux and bloating.

HERBAL INGREDIENTS

4 tablespoons aloe vera
   powder
4 tablespoons slippery elm
   bark powder
4 tablespoons
   marshmallow root
   powder

METHOD

Make the Herbal Powder base recipe (p. 33) with the herbal ingredients.

DOSAGE

1 heaped tablespoon in a full glass of water, to be taken up to three times daily before or after meals. Be sure to keep hydration up, drinking extra water to assist the passage of the powders through the gastrointestinal tract.

See Bloating Protocol (p. 148); Diarrhoea Protocol (p. 152)

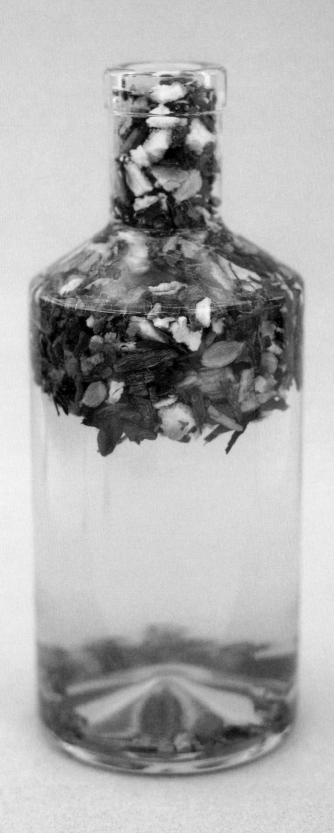

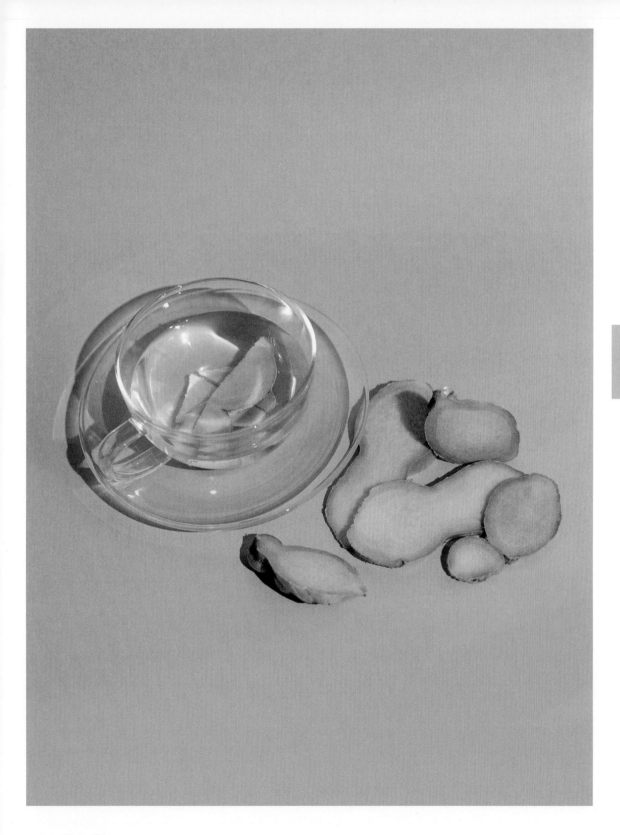

ABOVE *Ginger Tea*
OPPOSITE *Spiced Herbal Bitters*

Gut-Healing Smoothie

HERBAL INGREDIENTS

1 tablespoon **Gut-Healing Powder** (p. 165)

½ teaspoon turmeric rhizome powder or 1 teaspoon fresh turmeric rhizome

1 cup strong infused **Chamomile Tea** (p. 161)

1 teaspoon tremella powder (optional)

NUTRITIONAL INGREDIENTS

1–2 frozen bananas

2 tablespoons hemp seeds

1 tablespoon macadamia nut butter or nut butter of choice

a pinch of vanilla powder or a dash of vanilla extract

½ cup coconut water

1–2 teaspoons collagen powder (optional)

This delicious and digestively supportive concoction is a wonderful morning greeting for the gut. Smoothies are a great way to get in a dose of nutrient-dense goodness, with the added bonus of being very easily digested.

MAKES 1 SERVE

METHOD

Place all the ingredients in a blender and blend until well combined.

See Bloating Protocol (p. 148)

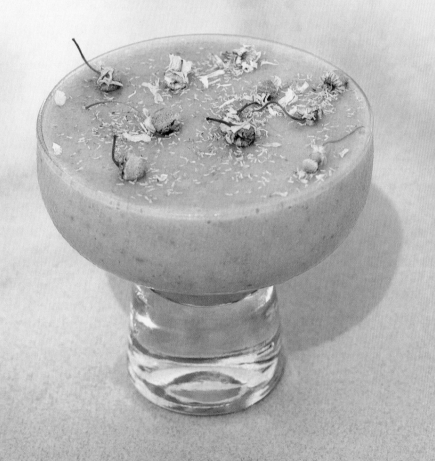

Mint Julep Oxymel

A fresh breath of minty goodness, perfect for nausea or to soothe digestive discomfort. This blend can be therapeutic or recreational – it makes a lovely garden-fresh spritzer when paired with sparkling water.

HERBAL INGREDIENTS

1 cup dried peppermint leaf
1 cup dried spearmint leaf

METHOD

Make the Oxymel base recipe (p. 34) with the herbal ingredients.

DOSAGE

Take as needed, but if belly symptoms are present, dose frequently as suggested in the dosing guidelines (p. 45).

See Nausea Protocol (p. 155)

Neutraliser Capsules

A superb synergistic formula to ease irritation of the gastrointestinal tract. Fitting for indigestion, reflux, discomfort and bloating. With key carminatives and demulcents, this encapsulated blend is here to harmonise symptoms and relieve gut woes.

HERBAL INGREDIENTS

½ tablespoon licorice root powder
½ tablespoon fennel seed powder
½ tablespoon meadowsweet powder
1 tablespoon slippery elm bark powder
½ tablespoon ginger rhizome powder

METHOD

Make the Capsules base recipe (p. 29) with the herbal ingredients.

DOSAGE

Depending on severity of symptoms, follow the dosages suggested in the dosing guidelines (p. 44).

See Indigestion protocol (p. 154)

Spiced Herbal Bitters

HERBAL INGREDIENTS

2 tablespoons dried
  gentian root
2 tablespoons dried
  dandelion root
2 tablespoons dried
  angelica root
2 tablespoons dried
  orange peel
2 tablespoons dried
  cinnamon chips
10 dried cardamom pods

An awakener of digestive juices, this earthy, warming combination of herbal bitters stimulates the appetite and aids digestion, powering the gut and banishing bloating. This blend also makes a perfect base for a celebratory cocktail!

METHOD

Make the Tincture base recipe (p. 38) with the herbal ingredients.

DOSAGE

1 teaspoon best taken 15–30 minutes before a meal or as needed, a maximum of three times daily.

See Bloating Protocol (p. 148)
See also Low Appetite (p. 172)

THE GUT

Rescue Remedies

HALITOSIS

Chew a few fennel seeds for fresh breath. With its high volatile-oil content creating an aromatic force-field, fennel offers sweet relief when you are experiencing bad breath. Choose fennel seeds for the win when combating oral odours – these seeds are laden with antimicrobial and antibacterial properties.

PS: Look to improve your overall gut health if bad breath persists.

LOW APPETITE

Stimulate your appetite with the **Spiced Herbal Bitters** (p. 171) or the **Botanical Bitters** (p. 157), best taken 15–30 minutes before a meal. Including more bitter greens in your diet (for example, rocket/arugula, bitter lettuces such as chicory and endive, and dandelion leaf) will also encourage digestive mechanisms to tick over and stimulate a suppressed appetite.

VOMITING

Super-simple **Ginger Tea** (p. 165) is a perfect queller of nausea and vomiting. If you are unable to keep liquids down, try chewing on a slice of fresh ginger root (or rhizome).

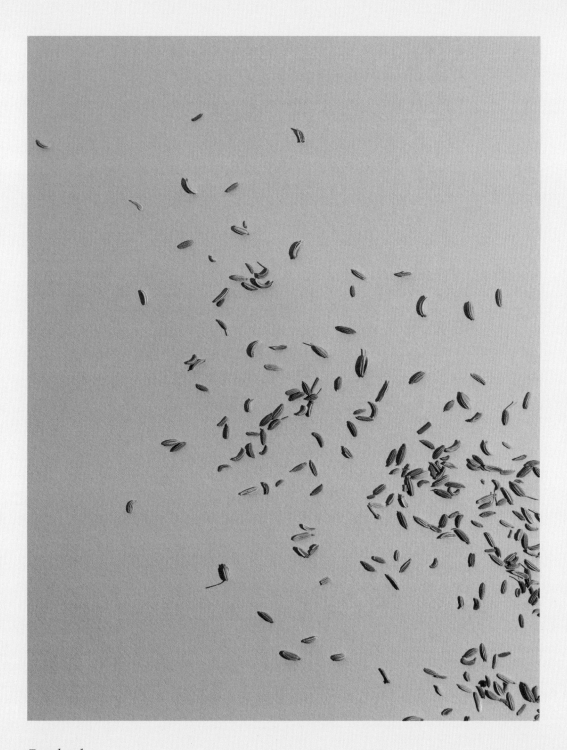

Fennel seeds

Hormone Health

Hormones are no joke. Any person who has experienced premenstrual syndrome (PMS), pregnancy or menopause will attest to the power that hormonal changes wield over us. They are also deeply complex; there are a plethora of hormones constantly circulating through our body's systems. A myriad of hormonal imbalances can present, from excessively oily skin, to mood dips, to missing menstrual cycles. These symptoms often indicate the need to rebalance hormonal health and to course-correct uncomfortable manifestations. Our hormonal health is ruled by the endocrine system: an overarching, highly intuitive 'control centre'. The endocrine system has many dutiful purposes, encompassing regulation of the metabolism, heart rate, appetite, sleep/wake cycle, stress response, body temperature, reproduction, menstruation and much more. The collection of glands responsible for these jobs comprise the hypothalamus, pituitary, pineal, thyroid, parathyroid and thymus, as well as the adrenals, ovaries, testes and pancreas. Given that our network of hormones spans multiple glands and organs, and impacts all systems of the body in one form or another, it is wise to look at hormonal health in a truly holistic manner.

If you are a person who bleeds monthly, or who historically has bled monthly, you will be familiar with your menstrual cycle: whether it keeps a perfect beat, like clockwork; whether it is painful for you; or whether it goes missing for extended periods of time. This cycle gives deeper insight into your body and being, and creates an invitation to get to know the inner workings of your own hormonal health.

The anatomy of the pelvis holds emotional layers that are often entangled in our body's precious sacral regions. These powerful yet tender centres hold stories and beliefs that often quite magically disrupt our menstrual cycles and create a held tension. In turn these held tensions create an echo through the subtle anatomies of the body, mind and spirit (energetic centres such as chakras and meridians) and can greatly impact hormonal harmony. It is so important to look at the energetic and emotional health of your body, not just the obvious layer of physical health.

Herbs have a marvellous way of communicating with your hormones.

Through a number of mechanisms, herbs can encourage a missing cycle to return or normalise, shift the quality of a menstrual bleed from barely there to an even flow, ease period pain and clear vaginal thrush.

Earthly angels, the plants are here to help.

Consider these the gateways to hormonal happiness

— I cannot stress enough the degree to which nutrition impacts our hormonal health. Harnessing the power of food as medicine is key to encouraging hormonal balance.

— Everyone has their own unique needs, but eating a varied, wholefoods diet (see p. 20) that covers your daily required intake of proteins, beneficial fats and complex carbohydrates is always a good thing. Ensure your meals are full to the brim with a diverse rainbow of veggies too, of course.

— Balancing your blood sugar is basically hormonal gospel! Pay attention to your relationship with nutrition choices and regularity of meals, and consider the **Sweet Treat Tea** (p. 201) if your sweet tooth is hard to say no to.

— Under-eating can also drastically impact your menstrual cycle, as can a low-carbohydrate diet. Be mindful of dietary fads and listen to your body – the wisest one of all.

— Patience is a virtue. When working to improve hormonal imbalances with plant medicines and natural interventions, expect three to four cycles (12–16 weeks) to pass before witnessing a shift.

HORMONE HEALTH

DAILY PROTOCOL

Boosting Fertility

Morning	Throughout the Day	
DRINK **The Pink Lady Tonic** (p. 196), a liver-loving adaptogenic blend that is a true pink-hued sensory delight. Schisandra berry, rose and beetroot powder create a harmonic experience while aiding the liver, softening stress and opening the heart. **SPOON** a dose of the **Iron-Lift Slow-Brew Syrup** (p. 60), to nourish and enrich the body. This blend cultivates vitality and internal strength, priming the body and its iron stores for creation.	**SIP** on a big pot of **You Are a Juicy Peach Tea** (p. 207), a fertility-enhancing and hormone-balancing blend. The name is more about the metaphor of a luscious, ripe fruit ready for the picking than it is about the actual fruit of the peach (which this recipe lacks!).	
Enhancements	**CONSIDER** the need for perspective. Once you have decided that you want to become a parent, it is usually hard to focus on anything else. Go gently with your process – babies seem to come earthside on their own unique timelines!	

There are so many factors that impact our fertility, and each individual case will be entirely unique. The good news is that natural interventions and herbal remedies have been employed to enhance fertility for aeons, and many have impressive efficacy in re-harmonising hormones, reducing stress and preparing the body for healthy conception. Focusing on nourishing your body and being is the most potent portal to enhancing creation mode!

Afternoon	Evening
SNACK on a few delicious **Maca Bliss Balls** (p. 67). An afternoon sweet treat to look forward to, the balls provide a nice dose of fertility-supportive, adaptogenic maca root. If any cycle irregularities are present, roll your Maca bliss balls in some seeds, in alignment with the **Seed Cycling** guidelines (p. 198) – super simple, and a great way to add some nice crunch.	**MASSAGE** over the lower pelvic and uterine area with **Womb Oil** (p. 206). This practice brings a sense of connection and self-love to the womb space, while nourishing happy hormones, and uterine and ovarian health.

HORMONE HEALTH

PRACTISE THE PILLARS

HYDRATE aplenty. Take care of your earthly vessel and spirit by eating **GOOD FOOD**. Softening your energy by prioritising **REST** can be a potent practice. Engage in daily **BODY MOVEMENT**, perhaps outdoors where you can **CONNECT WITH NATURE**. Stay vigilant about your personal, internal, **SELF-TALK**.

Irregular Cycles

Upon Rising	Throughout the Day	
DRINK a cup of **Dandy Coffee** (p. 186), to support liver function. This in turn balances hormonal health. Happily, this simple blend of dandelion root and chicory root will replace traditional coffee without the fallout that caffeine can create for hormonal health.	**EAT** seeds! **Seed Cycling** (p. 198) daily will encourage oestrogen and progesterone to rebalance. Essentially, this practice involves incorporating a small handful of seeds into your diet; they can be used in a smoothie, sprinkled over your breakfast of choice or added to snazz up a salad.	
Enhancements	**CONSIDER** that there are always underlying reasons for your cycle losing its balance. High stress, dietary changes, overexercising, thyroid issues and PCOS (polycystic ovary syndrome) can all be contributing factors.	

There can be many reasons for a missing or inconsistent period. Plant medicines are very clever at encouraging a cycle to return and remain in a monthly rhythm. They encourage the womb space to respond and hormone-receptor sites to sing; they also encourage thickening of the endometrium (lining) of the uterus, readying it to shed. If you are experiencing irregular cycles, try the herbal combos below.

Morning and Afternoon	Evening
DOSE UP on **The Loop Tincture** (p. 192), made with chaste tree, motherwort, calendula and dong quai. This herbal combo encourages healthful cycles and the return of your monthly bleed.	**STEAM** with a **Pelvic Steam** (p. 194), once or twice monthly, to embolden regularity of the menstrual cycle. This ancient practice involves (let me put it to you straight!) steaming the vagina with herbals. Vaginal tissues are incredibly absorbent. Steaming aids movement in cases of uterine stagnation and often yields a profound impact on cycle regulation. Do some research, and consider whether this is right for you.

PRACTISE THE PILLARS

They are all key factors in encouraging a regular cycle – bring them all on board. Eat really GOOD FOOD (as clean as possible). Commit to daily BODY MOVEMENT. Keep a strong, consistent focus on stress reduction.

HORMONE
HEALTH

DAILY PROTOCOL

Menopause

Morning	Throughout the Day	
POP the **Meno-Pause Capsules** (p. 193), a blended formula of beloved balancing herbs to fluidly assist the passage of change. This recipe is aimed at easing the common presentations of anxiety, sleeplessness and vaginal dryness experienced in menopause.	**DRESS** salads with the **Greens Vinegar** (p. 187), a simple, herbal, mineral-dense apple cider vinegar infusion. Rich in calcium to aid bone health (which is absolutely impacted by menopausal hormonal changes), this replenishing, sour bomb will happily adorn your green leaves and add absorbable minerals to your everyday. Another option is to take 1–3 tablespoons neat, daily. *and/or* **SIP** the **Nutritive Overnight Infusion** (p. 194). Deeply nourishing, and dense in minerals and vitamins, this deep jewel-green infusion adds hydration with a nutritive twist.	
Enhancements	**CONSIDER** black cohosh, one herb that is beyond appropriate for life's chapter leading into and spanning menopause. This can be taken in a tablet complex form and is quite readily available at health food stores.	

Menopause heralds a new chapter of womanhood, associated with the archetype of the 'crone' – a phase in life and experience that should garner honour and respect. The collective emphasis on the value of youthfulness has served to cast menopause in a fairly heinous light. Yet, if we could subvert the negative rhetoric and allow women's bodies to be in motion and in change, perhaps we could more confidently claim menopause as a sacred rite of passage! As the body shifts away from reproduction as its focus, there is a new balance to be found. It is super important to keep the adrenal system nourished and to be aware of the hormonal and metabolic changes happening in this cycle, with sleeplessness, hot flushes and weight gain rife. As the body shifts gears, we need to hold it a little more purposefully.

Morning and Afternoon	Evening
DRINK a strong brewed cup of **No Sweats Tea** (p. 193), to ward off hot flushes if present. Sage is a key player here, calming the common flushing experienced in menopause.	**DOSE UP** on the **Slumber Drops** (p. 69) before bed, if sleep is extra light and broken. With kava, reishi and rose, these drops will guide the way into restfulness. *or* **POP** The **Dream Duster** capsules (p. 58), or you can just add the powder directly into your warm, plant-based milk of choice, as an alternative remedy for light or broken sleep patterns. This sedative blend contains passionflower, skullcap and chamomile to lull you into the quiet of the night.

PRACTISE THE PILLARS

Stay well **HYDRATED**. Eat really **GOOD FOOD**. Allow yourself to truly **REST**. Claim space and peacefulness wherever possible. Move your beautiful body. Listen to internal **SELF-TALK**, go gently, come from the heart. **CONNECT WITH NATURE**, witness how she changes and transforms, just like you.

HORMONE HEALTH

PMS (Premenstrual Syndrome)

Throughout the Day	Evening
EAT seeds, by practising **Seed Cycling** (p. 198) to balance hormones and aid in the reduction of PMS symptoms. This simple, down-to-earth practice involves adding flax seeds and pumpkin seeds to your diet on the follicular phase of the menstrual cycle (days 1–14), and then rotating to sesame and sunflower seeds in the luteal phase of the cycle (days 14–28). Eat these seeds as a topping on your porridge or sprinkled over salads, or simply add them to a smoothie. **SPOON** a dose of the **Uplifting Oxymel** (p. 205), to cocoon and soothe your tenderness, irritability and tension. With St John's wort, tulsi and borage, this bright-hearted blend brings much-needed relief.	**SIP** on a pot of **Harmonising Hormones Tea** (p. 188), to invoke the gentleness within. This blend is laden with hormone-balancing herbs – chaste tree, peony and shatavari – paired with the softness of rose and the nourishing goodness of nettle, red clover and peppermint to reduce tension. Best drunk daily when you are actively working on hormone balancing. **FLOAT** in a warm bath infused with **Herbal Magnesium Bath Soak** (p. 191). There really is nothing more therapeutic than immersing your body in warm water with cheerful flowers bopping around. Flowers and leaves add aromatic elements for pain reduction and mood elevation. This is an uplifting practice of joyful self-nurture – with the added bonus of magnesium-rich Epsom salts to ease PMS symptoms and wash away tension.

Hormones can go bananas, and anyone who has a menstrual cycle will attest to the hold that PMS can have over them. The governing symptoms of PMS include sore, tender breasts; irritability; weight gain; anxiety and nervous tension; mood swings; heightened emotional states and sensitivity; skin breakouts; an insatiable appetite; headaches; a sore back ... the list goes on. Fortunately, the following protocol offers many dynamic healers to soften the sharp edges before your bleed arrives.

Enhancements

PRACTISE THE PILLARS

BODY MOVEMENT is an important piece to alleviate PMS. Combine this with **CONNECTING WITH NATURE** – a brisk walk outdoors or a jog can bring sweet relief.

Bodacious Breast Oil

HERBAL INGREDIENTS

¼ cup dried violet leaf

¼ cup dried calendula
flowers

¼ cup dried yarrow
flowers/leaf

¼ cup dried burdock root

*Note: Breast tissue begins
below the collarbone,
extending to the mid-section
of the ribs, over the breast and
underneath the arm.*

There simply is not enough information out there around the importance of breast massage, so I am delighted to bring your attention to the following recipe to encourage this practice! This herbal-infused oil is laced with lymphatic-supportive plants, which aid the flow of lymphatic fluids in the breast tissues in the upper chest region, encouraging drainage and detoxification. Lather on this oil-based skin food for a potent, nourishing practice that reconnects you with your beautiful body.

METHOD

Make the Herbal-Infused Oil base recipe (p. 31) with the herbal ingredients.

DOSAGE

This is an anytime practice – simply drop a teaspoon of oil into your palm and begin to cover the chest area with the oil. Start at the nipple, massaging in upward circles and moving towards the armpit with upward strokes.

See Breast Health (p. 208)

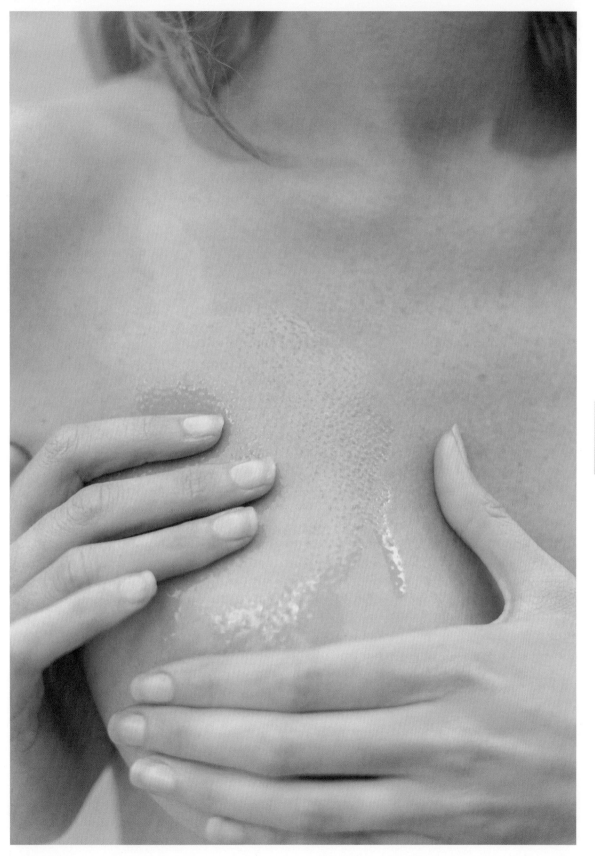

Dandelion Leaf Tea

Nutritive dandelion leaf offers a gentle diuretic action, perfect to combat puffiness, stimulate fluid retention and encourage excess fluid movement.

HERBAL INGREDIENT

2 teaspoons dried
  dandelion leaf

METHOD

Make the Medicinal Tea base recipe (p. 33) with the dandelion leaf.

See Fluid Retention (p. 208)

Dandy Coffee

Full transparency: this recipe has absolutely nothing to do with coffee, besides the fact that dandelion root makes a wonderful alternative! Here, it is combined with prebiotic and gut-loving chicory root. With a bitter, aromatic taste and a deep-brown hue, this brew is by far the best option when you are seeking a non-caffeinated beverage that can still hold up well with a splash of milk. Dandelion root is also wonderful for the liver.

HERBAL INGREDIENTS

2 teaspoons dried
  dandelion root
2 teaspoons dried chicory
  root

Note: For ease this blend can also be made as a medicinal tea. However, in order to extract optimal medicinal benefits from the dried root, it is best prepared as a decoction.

METHOD

Make the Decoction base recipe (p. 29) with the herbal ingredients and add your milk of choice!

See Irregular Cycles Protocol (p. 178)

Ginger Poultice

Bring warmth, and ease pain and cramping, with a simple ginger-root poultice. Super helpful for menstrual pain, digestive cramping and arthritic pain.

HERBAL INGREDIENT

2 tablespoons fresh ginger rhizome or 1 tablespoon dried ginger powder

METHOD

Mix your ginger with a little hot water to create a paste and follow the Poultice base recipe (p. 36). Be sure to use the two-cloth 'sandwich' technique mentioned in the base recipe.

See Menstrual Cramps (p. 209)

HORMONE HEALTH

Greens Vinegar

A jewel-green delight that you can use to dress your salads, add to your sparkling water or spoon straight on in for a chlorophyll-laden, plant-rich hit! This is a super-simple herbal recipe, encouraging you to utilise plants growing nearby (be sure to master your edible plant identification) or those you may be keeping in dried form in your herbal apothecary. Dandelion leaves are a great place to start, and would be a happy choice either as the sole ingredient or as an add-on in a medley of vibrant greens.

HERBAL INGREDIENTS

1 cup fresh or ½ cup dried dandelion leaf, gotu kola leaf, plantago leaf, nettle leaf, violet leaf (and so on)

METHOD

Make the Vinegar base recipe (p. 39) with the herbal ingredients.

See Menopause Protocol (p. 180)

Harmonising Hormones Tea

Encourage happy hormones with this lady-loving blend, full of supportive, woman-centric herbals. Shatavari, peony and chaste tree nourish and normalise a healthful menstrual cycle, while nettle and red clover add key nutritive elements for a fortified body and being. Notes of peppermint and rose soften the sip. Brew this blend strongly.

HERBAL INGREDIENTS

1 teaspoon dried peony root

1 ½ teaspoons dried chaste tree berries

2 teaspoons dried shatavari root

2 teaspoons dried rose petals/buds

1 teaspoon dried nettle leaf

2 teaspoons dried peppermint leaf

2 teaspoons dried red clover flowers

METHOD

Make the Medicinal Tea base recipe (p. 33) with the herbal ingredients.

See PMS Protocol (p. 182)

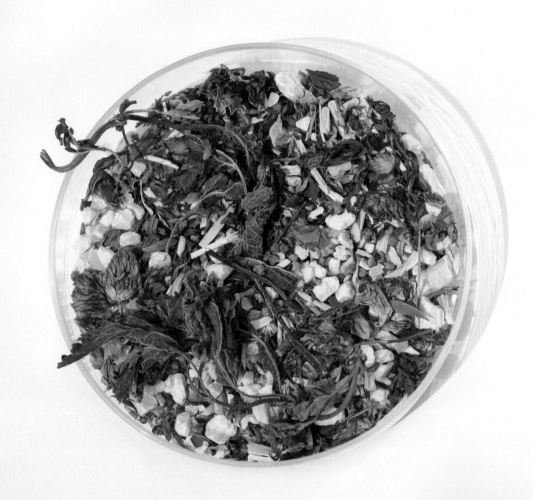

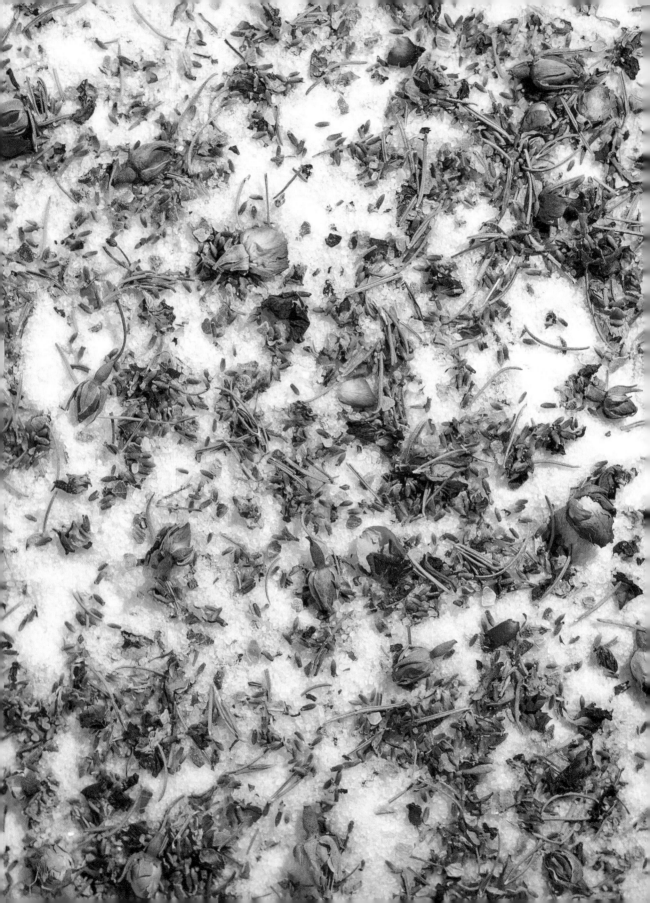

Herbal Magnesium Bath Soak

HERBAL INGREDIENTS

3 tablespoons dried
    rosemary
2 tablespoons dried rose
    petals/rosebuds
4 tablespoons dried
    lavender
2 tablespoons dried lemon
    peel
1 ½ cups Epsom salts
1 ½ tablespoons olive oil

Note: Be sure to drink plenty of water after your bath, as Epsom salts activate clearance of toxins. This soak is best taken in the evening, followed by an early night's sleep.

The most beautiful and medicinal bath soak for a lingering headache, tension and muscular aches. If you do not have access to a bath, make this into a foot bath! Our feet are often neglected, although they do such important work holding our bodies in presence and anchoring us to the earth. Now and then they need extra TLC, and this bath is the perfect remedy to relax the muscles and unlock tension in the body. You can absolutely get interpretive with this blend, utilising any fragrant herbs you have handy to assist the body, mind and spirit to deeply unwind. This recipe also looks beyond beautiful and makes the most thoughtful gift!

METHOD

Add all the ingredients to a running bath.

Alternatively, for a foot-soak version, halve the quantity of each of the nominated ingredients and add them to a large round basin or a bucket filled with warm water.

Submerge your body in the bath or submerge your feet in the infused water and soak up the serenity for 20 minutes or so. You can supercharge this practice with a relaxing meditation or by listening to soothing music.

Dry your body and feet thoroughly and gently, drain your bath water, and compost your spent bath herbs.

See PMS Protocol (p. 182)

HORMONE HEALTH

Lighten the Flow Tincture

When the menstrual cycle is heavy and blood loss is marked, this astringent and antispasmodic tincture can be brought on board to ease the pain and discomfort associated with dysmenorrhoea. This is a key blend to have in the home apothecary, to call on as needed to soften an uncomfortable menstrual cycle.

HERBAL INGREDIENTS

¼ cup dried yarrow
   flowers/leaf
¼ cup dried shepherd's
   purse stem/flowers/leaf
¼ cup dried cinnamon
   bark
½ cup dried raspberry leaf

METHOD

Make the Tincture base recipe (p. 38) with the herbal ingredients.

See Dysmenorrhoea (p. 208)

The Loop Tincture

If your menstrual-cycle loop is out of whack, this is the tincture to prep. Hormones are truly complex, and there are myriad reasons why your cycle may be overactive in nature (painful, heavy bleeds), underactive in nature (scanty, light bleeds) or entirely missing in action. This tincture combo works with key herbals to regulate the menstrual cycle.

HERBAL INGREDIENTS

½ cup dried chaste tree
   berries
¼ cup dried motherwort
   leaf/flowers/stem
¼ cup dried calendula
   flowers
¼ cup dried dong quai
   root/leaf

METHOD

Make the Tincture base recipe (p. 38) with the herbal ingredients.

DOSAGE

Be sure to check whether these herbals suit your symptom picture, and work with their medicine for a committed period of time – ideally a minimum of 3 months for sustained change.

See Irregular Cycles Protocol (p. 178)
See also Scanty, Light Period (p. 209)

Meno-Pause Capsules

Mood lifters, nootropics, adaptogens and hormone balancers are all woven throughout this formula. So very helpful for symptoms commonly experienced in menopause, such as vaginal dryness, sleeplessness and anxiety. These herbal capsules work to support this chapter of change, and mitigate the often-challenging symptoms.

HERBAL INGREDIENTS

½ tablespoon black
  cohosh powder
½ tablespoon dong quai
  powder
½ tablespoon motherwort
  powder
½ tablespoon lemon balm
  powder
¼ tablespoon licorice
  powder
½ tablespoon spirulina
  powder
¼ tablespoon burdock
  powder

METHOD

Make the Capsules base recipe (p. 29) with the herbal ingredients.

See Menopause Protocol (p. 180)

HORMONE HEALTH

No Sweats Tea

Hot flushes are a common symptom of hormonal changes in menopause and are an often-petulant presentation – uncomfortable, sudden and disarming! This formula relies heavily on the powers of wise sage leaf, with its inherent ability to calm flushing severity and frequency. Brew strongly and sip often to quell internal heat waves.

HERBAL INGREDIENTS

1 teaspoon dried sage
1 teaspoon dried yarrow
  flowers/leaf
2 teaspoons dried
  spearmint leaf

METHOD

Make the Medicinal Tea base recipe (p. 33) with the herbal ingredients.

See Menopause Protocol (p. 180)

Nutritive Overnight Infusion

This hydrating union of strengthening herbals – imbued with red clover, oat straw, nettle and alfalfa, and rich in minerals and vitamins – helps you to increase daily nutrition with ease. Nettle lends a force-field of adrenal support, and oat straw sympathetically soothes the nerves. Squeeze a little lemon in for extra tang, and a dash of honey to add sweetness if desired.

HERBAL INGREDIENTS

1 tablespoon dried oat
straw or milky oat tops
1 tablespoon dried nettle
leaf
1 tablespoon dried alfalfa
leaf
1 tablespoon dried red
clover flowers

METHOD

Make the Overnight Water Infusion base recipe (p. 34) with the herbal ingredients.

See Menopause Protocol (p. 180)

Pelvic Steam

In cultures worldwide, we have long steamed the vagina! This practice is particularly helpful for those with sluggish or missing menstrual cycles, encouraging tissue nourishment, blood circulation and healing. Pelvic steams can be an incredibly relaxing and transcendent self-care ritual. Steaming is suitable for many presentations, from postpartum healing to boosting fertility and much in between, but please be sure to do your research and look into whether a pelvic steam suits your individual needs.

HERBAL INGREDIENTS

2 tablespoons dried
mugwort leaf
2 tablespoons dried lady's
mantle
2 tablespoons dried
motherwort leaf/flowers/
stem
2 tablespoons dried
rosebuds
2 tablespoons dried red
clover flowers
2 tablespoons dried
hawthorn berries

METHOD

Create a calm quiet space for this practice. Add serene elements, such as meditative music or your favourite scented candle.

In a large saucepan, add your dried herbal ingredients and 12 cups of water. Bring to a boil over high heat and simmer over medium heat for 10 minutes.

Note: The practice of pelvic steaming has absolutely nothing to do with cleaning the vagina. The vagina really is a wondrous, self-cleaning mechanism.

Cautionary notes: Never steam when you are pregnant or possibly pregnant, or when you have your period. Avoid steaming if you have an active internal or external infection, or if you have an IUD.

If you are working deeply on a hormonal issue, it really is best to consult a practitioner (herbalist or well-versed plant-wise midwife) to get some customised care and support with steaming.

Remove from the heat. Strain out the herbs with a fine-mesh sieve (and compost your spent plant material).

Pour the infused hot water into a large heatproof bowl. To avoid any incidental burns when steaming, do not pour the infused water back into the large saucepan. Cover the heatproof bowl promptly to trap the steam, and take it into your quiet location of choice.

Place the bowl on the floor and remove the lid.

You MUST test the steam with your hand first. If it is too hot, allow it to cool.

Once the steam is at a comfortable temperature, get undressed from the waist down. Position your legs either side of the steamy bowl, and wrap a towel around your waist to create a steam tent of sorts.

Remain standing, kneeling or seated above the bowl for as long as it feels good: aim for 15–30 minutes maximum. Utilise this time to be still with yourself. Meditate, breathe and connect.

When you have completed your steam, discard the steam water.

Go gently, stay hydrated and get to bed early.

DOSAGE

Generally, steaming can be undertaken once or twice monthly, but please avoid the week of menstruation.

See Irregular Cycles Protocol (p. 178)

The Pink Lady Tonic

HERBAL INGREDIENTS

½ teaspoon schisandra
    berry powder
½ teaspoon rose petal
    powder
½ teaspoon beetroot
    powder
½ teaspoon vanilla bean
    powder

*Note: Adding a sweet
spoonful of honey is highly
recommended.*

Drinking something pink always feels extra delightful (are you with me on this one?!), and this tonic embodies the radical vibration offered by such a brilliant colour. Three distinct, pink-hued plants combine to assist the liver, open the heart and soothe internal stress. With adaptogenic schisandra berry, liver-loving beetroot, and rose to ignite self-love, this milky tonic is wonderful warm or totally lovely over ice.

METHOD

Make the Plant Mylk Tonic base recipe (p. 35) with the herbal ingredients.

See Boosting Fertility Protocol (p. 176)

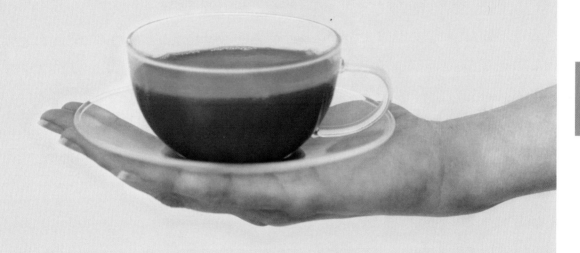

Seed Cycling

DAYS 1–14:
FOLLICULAR PHASE

1–2 tablespoons ground
   pumpkin seeds
1–2 tablespoons ground
   flax seeds

DAYS 14–28:
LUTEAL PHASE

1–2 tablespoons ground
   sesame seeds
1–2 tablespoons ground
   sunflower seeds

Using seed cycling to balance the menstrual cycle is a beloved naturopathic practice. When there are imbalances within the menstrual cycle, symptoms such as PMS, sore breasts, skin breakouts, irregular or painful periods, weight gain and anxiety may present. Seed cycling is a really helpful daily practice and is ideal for those coming off the oral contraceptive pill or seeking to rebalance a missing cycle.

HOW TO SEED CYCLE

Menstruation is governed by two distinct cycles: the first 14 days represent the follicular phase (onset of menstruation to ovulation), and the last 14 days the luteal phase (ovulation to menstruation). In the follicular phase, oestrogen rises; in the luteal phase, progesterone will be the rising force. In the follicular phase, pumpkin and flax seeds work to harmonise oestrogen and promote the production of progesterone, and in the luteal phase sunflower and sesame seeds offer key nutrients to support progesterone. These seeds are full of essential plant-rich nutrients, fatty acids, and minerals and vitamins – all of which help hormones to regain their balance.

Seed cycling can be synchronised with the lunar cycle to help establish a rhythm in the menstrual cycle: follicular-phase seeds should be taken in the time between the new moon and full moon, and luteal-phase seeds taken in the time between the full moon and new moon. The moon is quite a mighty force – menstrual cycles often naturally synchronise with a moon cycle, with bleeds often experienced on either the new or full moon.

You can purchase the seeds already ground, or you can grind your own. I recommend grinding your own to ensure freshness. You can do this in a blender or a spice grinder.

This is a daily practice, so finding ways to get these seeds into your diet is the main challenge. There are plenty of imaginative, easy ways to weave them in: try adding your seeds to smoothies, porridge, granola, soups, salads, chia pudding, bliss balls or yoghurt.

Stick with this practice for at least 3–6 months to encourage a healthful cycle.

See Boosting Fertility Protocol (p. 176); Irregular Cycles Protocol (p. 178); PMS Protocol (p. 182)

HORMONE
HEALTH

Soften the Sacral Tea

HERBAL INGREDIENTS

3 teaspoons dried ginger
  rhizome

2 teaspoons dried wild
  yam root

1 teaspoon dried cramp
  bark

1 teaspoon dried chaste
  tree berries

4 teaspoons dried fennel
  seeds

Bring sweet relief to menstrual cramping with this supportive tisane, full of antispasmodic and anodyne-rich herbals to calm tidal waves of pelvic discomfort. If you often suffer with painful bleeds and cramping, bring this blend on board 4 days prior to the onset of your menstrual cycle and continue to sip daily throughout your cycle. Keep a pot on the stove in times of need, simmering this grounded, root-rich blend when needed.

METHOD

Make the Decoction base recipe (p. 29) with the herbal ingredients. This is a potent brew! As such, it is wise to dilute it with extra water and add a little honey for a smoother taste.

DOSAGE

When cramps are heightened, be sure to follow the acute dosing guidelines (p. 44).

See Dysmenorrhoea (p. 208); Menstrual Cramps (p. 209)

Sweet Treat Tea

HERBAL INGREDIENTS

3 teaspoons dried
   cinnamon bark
1 teaspoon dried ginger
   rhizome
1 teaspoon dried licorice
   root

Bust sugar cravings with the help of this scrumptious tea! Licorice root is a natural sweetener, and notes of cosy cinnamon and ginger float gently through the blend – all working to curb your sweet tooth and balance blood sugar. This enhances utilisation of glucose in the body, a super-helpful action when you are seeking to self-regulate the longing for sweet treats.

METHOD

Make the Decoction base recipe (p. 29) or Medicinal Tea base recipe (p. 33) with the herbal ingredients.

See Balanced Blood Sugar (p. 208)

HORMONE
HEALTH

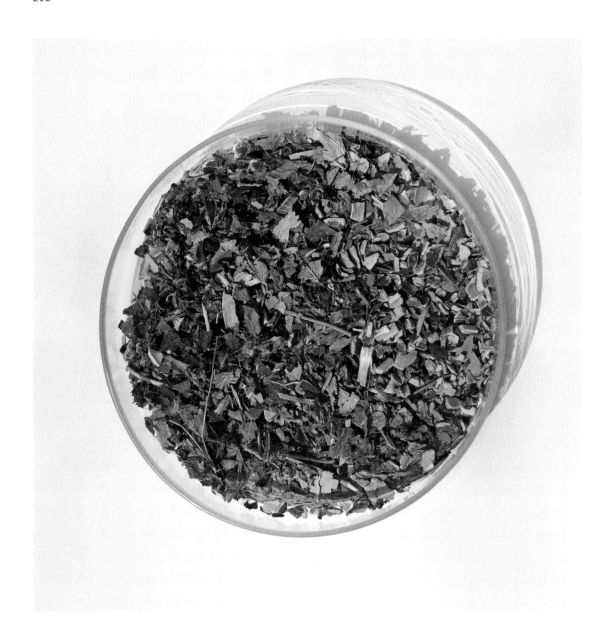

Soften the Sacral Tea

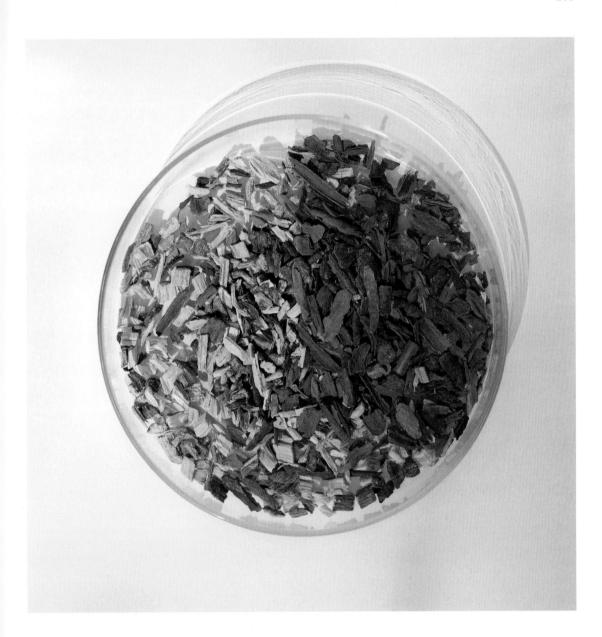

Sweet Treat Tea

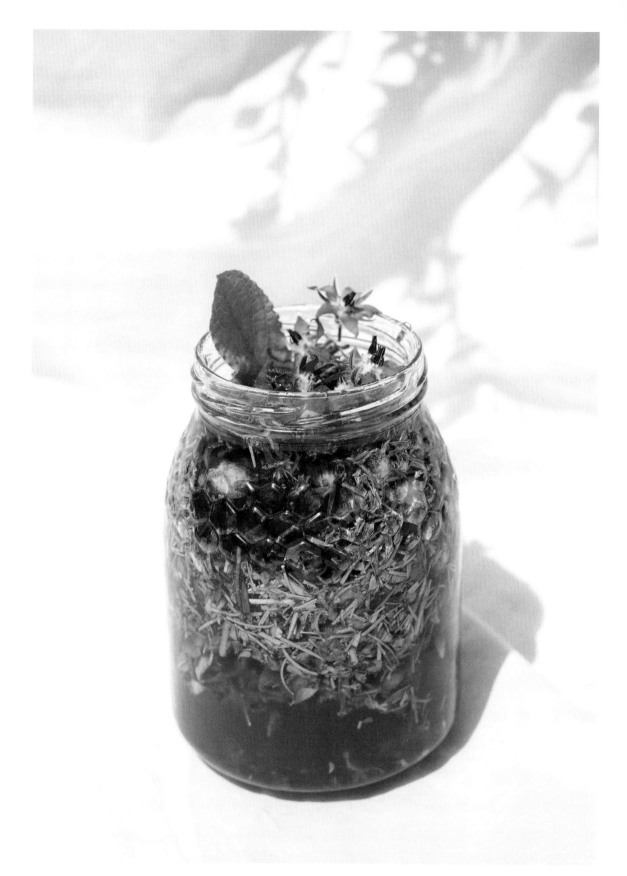

Uplifting Oxymel

HERBAL INGREDIENTS

¾ cup dried or 1 ½ cup fresh St John's wort leaf/flowers

¼ cup dried or ½ cup fresh borage flowers

½ cup dried rosemary leaf/flowers

½ cup dried rose petals

¾ cup dried tulsi leaf/flowers

Note: I have given a fresh plant material option in this recipe for a couple of the herbs that I feel work really well when used fresh, compared with dried. Feel free to blend fresh with dried plant material.

When internal clouds are heavy and there is no blue sky to be seen, this plant medicine is the most fitting remedy, a gentle offering working to soften depression and heaviness. Mood-enhancing herbs are married together here to create a celestial ambrosia of sorts, deliciously soaked in a golden-nectared oxymel base of honey and apple cider vinegar. The plants shall part the clouds and awaken the sunshine within you!

METHOD

Make the Oxymel base recipe (p. 34) with the herbal ingredients.

DOSAGE

Give this blend a go for a good period of time: 6 or more weeks, ideally, if you are experiencing a very low mood. I find that working with this blend for a prolonged period really allows the plants to work deeply to support and catalyse changes within.

See PMS Protocol (p. 182)

See also Depression Protocol (p. 274)

HORMONE HEALTH

Womb Oil

HERBAL INGREDIENTS

¼ cup dried motherwort
   leaf
¼ cup dried calendula
   flowers
¼ cup dried yarrow leaf/
   flowers
¼ cup dried ginger
   rhizome
¼ cup dried rose petals

*Note: Some find it advisable
to avoid womb massage when
menstruating and ovulating, as
it feels a little too stimulating.*

The womb space holds a wealth of power within. We often disregard the innate power emanating from our sacrums. A wonderful way to connect with the uterine area is with herbal oil massage. This grounding and deeply nurturing practice aids hormonal imbalances, assists fertility by supporting the reproductive organs, and encourages uterine circulation and tissue softening. Be mindful of self-talk and intention when connecting with this deeply personal practice.

METHOD

Make the Herbal-Infused Oil base recipe (p. 31) with the herbal ingredients.

Get comfy and lay down in your chosen cosy space. Drop a teaspoon of oil into the palm of your hand and create warmth by rubbing your hands together. Start to gently rub your lower abdomen (begin just under the belly button), reaching just to the top of the pubic bone, using gentle, circular, clockwise movements. Next, use downward strokes, massaging towards the pubic bone. Finish with gentle upward strokes. You can bring this practice down to the calves and into the feet to ground the body, or even up into the jaw. All parts of your body are connected, go where you feel called to – use your sage intuition!

DOSAGE

If you are actively calling in conception, welcome in this practice from the fourth day of menstruation to the day before ovulation.

See Boosting Fertility Protocol (p. 176)

You Are a Juicy Peach Tea

HERBAL INGREDIENTS

2 teaspoons dried chaste
tree berries

2 teaspoons dried dong
quai root

2 teaspoons dried
rehmannia root

3 teaspoons dried
cinnamon bark

2 teaspoons dried
shatavari root

4 teaspoons dried ginger
rhizome

2 teaspoons dried orange
peel

2 teaspoons dried licorice
root

Peaches are the fruits of fertility – luscious, fleshy and juicy. This slow-simmered tea embodies and emboldens the energy of ripeness within, harmonising hormonal health and encouraging fertility with a fusion of stellar plants. Shatavari (*Asparagus racemosus*) is a key tonic for female reproductive health and merges with some of the most revered potent fertility supporters in this beautiful blend.

METHOD

Make the Decoction base recipe (p. 29) with the herbal ingredients.

DOSAGE

Keep up this blend on a daily basis if you are actively working on fertility enhancement. Follow the dosage suggestions given in the dosing guidelines (p. 44).

See Boosting Fertility Protocol (p. 176)
See also Scanty, Light Period (p. 209)

HORMONE
HEALTH

Rescue Remedies

BALANCED BLOOD SUGAR

As mentioned throughout the whole hormonal health section, it is of the utmost importance to balance your blood sugar for steady, happy, healthy hormones – and for happy health in general. There are many herbs that will encourage even blood sugar and guard against a hypoglycaemic (low blood sugar) episode, working alongside good nutrition (essential!) to ward off repetitive sugar cravings. Bring on the **Sweet Treat Tea** (p. 201), an easy-to-drink blend dotted with cinnamon and licorice to satisfy your candy-craving tooth.

BREAST HEALTH

We often overlook the nurture and importance of breast health. A great way to support breast tissues and to encourage lymphatic flow is to practise self-massage using the **Bodacious Breast Oil** (p. 184), a herbal combo infused in oil. Breast tissue, fatty in nature, really appreciates topical oil applications. Welcome in this potent self-love practice weekly or twice weekly, to support hormonal health, discourage lumps and bumps, and activate lymphatic drainage.

DYSMENORRHOEA

When a menstrual bleed becomes very heavy, it can be incredibly draining and tiresome for the body and being. Be sure to try the **Lighten the Flow Tincture** (p. 192), with astringent herbs at the helm to ease associated discomfort and encourage a lighter flow. Sip on **Soften the Sacral Tea** (p. 200) throughout the day, to calm any cramping that is present.

PS: It is super common to experience an occasional, one-off heavier cycle. But if your cycle always presents on the noticeably heavy side, please be sure to consult with your healthcare practitioner to rule out fibroids, endometriosis and iron deficiency/anaemia; the latter is very common in menstruating women due to monthly blood loss. If so, add in a daily dose of the Iron-Lift Slow-Brew Syrup (p. 60).

FLUID RETENTION

Particularly around ovulation and throughout the onset or duration of menstruation, fluid retention is a not-so-lovely, but commonly experienced, symptom. Feeling puffy and bloated can put a serious dampener on your day. Try a super-simple pot of **Dandelion Leaf Tea** (p. 186), a potassium-rich, natural diuretic, to de-puff and encourage fluid flow.

MENSTRUAL CRAMPS

Menstrual cramps have the ability to derail all plans, and commonly demand a grin-and-bear-it approach through uncomfortable spasms, contractions and stabbing uterine sensations. Luckily there are many natural remedies we can employ to soften the tidal waves of cramping if need be. Ginger is a very helpful anti-inflammatory herb for menstrual cramps, working particularly well as a warming poultice. Pop on the **Ginger Poultice** (p. 187), an easy-to-make topical therapy, to ease painful cramping. Sip **Soften the Sacral Tea** (p. 200), a blend of cramp bark, fennel, chaste tree, motherwort and more. This formula works to ease severity of cramping and support a smoother cycle. If pain is incredibly severe, try the analgesic-rich **Sweet Relief Tincture** (p. 303).

PS: Magnesium in supplement form can be an essential ally in weathering menstrual cramps with a little more ease. A great-quality supplement rich in omega-3 and fatty acids (such as a fish oil) can support overall reduction of inflammation positively and contribute to a reduction of menstrual pain.

SCANTY, LIGHT PERIOD

If lighter periods are your norm, that is absolutely perfect, but if you are experiencing lighter flow randomly and consistently it can often indicate a hormonal imbalance, or perhaps is a signal that stress is taking its toll. Try **The Loop Tincture** (p. 192) or **You Are a Juicy Peach Tea** (p. 207) daily to inspire a wholesome full bleed.

VAGINAL THRUSH

Imbalances in vaginal flora can cause troublesome symptoms and discomfort. Thrush can be acute, coming and going quickly, or it can linger, with multiple flare-ups occurring. Although there are many more complex herbal vaginal suppositories, for ease try a (thoroughly unpleasant-sounding!) garlic clove inserted into the vagina. The only preparation needed is to peel the clove and pierce it with a knife, just a little nick, to release the inner medicine that supports vaginal bacterial health and eradicates irritation. You can create an easy exit plan by sewing a thread through the garlic clove; that way, you'll have no difficulty removing the clove, and there won't be any chance of it getting lost. Leave the clove inserted overnight and remove in the morning. You may have to repeat for a few nights.

PS: Changing your diet to eradicate all sugars is an important piece in healing vaginal thrush, which is caused by an overgrowth of the yeast Candida albicans. Following a no-sugar eating plan, with low intake of grains and starches, can be a very supportive practice. Eradicating alcohol is also essential to overcome acute and chronic thrush episodes. Remember that the vaginal microbiome is connected to the gut microbiome, so working on gut health is essential.

HORMONE HEALTH

Mums and Bubs

This delicate life chapter has long been a space where herbs have been employed. In the West, we have become extremely conservative with our cautions around plant medicines for pregnant people; I have been asked an incredible number of times whether it is safe to drink **Raspberry Leaf Tea** (p. 230) during a pregnancy.

It is, of course, enormously important to be vigilant about what you ingest during pregnancy. But it is also important to understand that plant medicines do not act like pharmaceuticals in the body.

Doing much less, herbwise, is a good rule of thumb to follow during pregnancy. Many plant medicines have cautions around pregnancy and lactation, so it is important to consult a solid herbal materia medica before ingesting medicinal plants. Go very softly with supplements – and please, be sure to always do your research and ask questions of your herbalist, naturopath, medical provider or midwife (who will often be versed in herbs, if more holistically minded in general).

The herculean undertaking – and marvel – of creation demands a lot of the body and being. Giving your body over to baby-making, and birthing and nourishing a little human, is a mammoth task, one that demands extra support and attention.

Many women do not foresee the depths of exhaustion into which postnatal depletion can lead them, nor the emotional weight that breastfeeding challenges may bring. As mothers and babies navigate the spectrum of entrenched concerns, there are always ways to bring plant medicines in to assist, to metaphorically swaddle and lullaby you and your little one as you find the way back to balance.

Infants, in their fresh incarnation of life, often need very little intervention with plant medicines overall. But there are a few really important herb-dense remedies to keep in your herbal first aid kit for things like teething and reflux. These seemingly minor issues can bring new parents to their knees, and the good news is that the plants are here to help.

A sweet side note

We must approach this subject with loving caution. It is laced with tenderness and sensitivity. We should be mindful of bringing sincere gentleness to our interactions with those who are experiencing the challenges of pregnancy, birthing and parenting, as well as dealing with their own sleep-deprived struggles. When we hold awareness, we can offer support.

Fortified Pregnancy Support

For Immunity

Immunity goes on a rollercoaster ride during pregnancy; some elements of the system are enhanced, while other elements are suppressed. Bring on the **Echinacea Tincture** (p. 101), beginning with a drop dose and increasing the amount to a more therapeutic dose as needed. This is particularly helpful in the cooler months, when it is common for a cold to loom, or when you may simply feel the general need to strengthen immunity.

Consider supplementation: Supplements such as vitamin C, zinc and lactoferrin are all indicated and safe at specific dosages. Please follow the RDA (recommended dietary allowance – that is, the recommended daily intake level) for dosage limitations.

For Morning Sickness

Sip on **Ginger Tea** (p. 165). Ginger is an incredible ally for combating nausea and is generally very effective.

A few tips: Eat smaller, more frequent, nutritious meals; consider a B6 supplement; hydrate; learn acupressure points for nausea relief; and counteract stress with mindfulness practice.

I truly do understand that researching herbals – safe or cautioned – for use during pregnancy can be a completely confusing process. There are many differing opinions! Keep it super simple and stripped back with this selection of herbals, to be used as needed. I also offer you solid clarity on the use of raspberry leaf in pregnancy. This protocol is a little different from the others, offering insight into an 'as needed' approach rather than a daily guide.

For Birth Preparation and Nourishment

Raspberry Leaf Tea (p. 230) has long been used to tone, strengthen and prep the uterus for birth. Historically, this plant medicine has been used in all stages of a pregnancy, but it is now more commonly suggested that women begin taking the tea at around 32 weeks pregnant. Start by drinking 1 cup daily and gradually increase to 3 cups daily in the final weeks before birthing. If you want to fancy this tea up and add extra nourishment, mix in equal parts oat straw and rosehips.

The flip side: I must offer the perspective that many herbalists in our modern day still value raspberry leaf as a very safe herb for use throughout a whole pregnancy. They believe its use will actually prevent miscarriage – rather than overly stimulating the uterus, as is commonly feared. If you have done your research and you want to work with this uber-nourishing plant, stick with these suggested doses: 1 cup daily in the first trimester, 2 cups daily in the second trimester and 3 cups daily in the third trimester.

MUMS AND BUBS

DAILY PROTOCOL

Lactation Support

Morning and Evening	Throughout the Day
### DROP	### DRINK
the **Mama Nourish Elixir** (p. 228) onto the tongue for a nutrifying lift. This delectable jammy formula offers gentle yet poignant nervous-system support for a weary, stressed mother. It is packed full of high-vibey (and safe-for-breastfeeding) herbs, alongside key galactagogue herbals to assist with a plentiful milk flow.	3–6 cups of the **Lactation Flow-Support Tea** (p. 226), chock full of medicinal plants to stimulate and hearten breast-milk production. This blend also tastes lovely iced, so if your brewed teapot has been neglected, no worries at all, keep sipping away.
	### SNACK
	on a few **Milkshake Bliss Balls** (p. 229). These creamy, plant-based, energy-dense bombs offer sustained energy support and encourage favourable milk flow.

Breastfeeding makes huge demands on the body. Sometimes this process flows with ease, and other times it does not, often creating an incredibly stressful experience for mum and bub. This protocol is rich in galactagogue herbs, to encourage milk flow.

Enhancements

PRACTISE THE PILLARS

HYDRATE aplenty – your body is giving so much liquid over when breastfeeding. Drink lots of water and herbal tea, as above. Do not forget to eat **GOOD FOOD**. It is common for a mama to let her own needs slip away, but you must be nourished in order to care for your bub. When stress looms, practise connecting with your breath to centre the body. Step outside to **CONNECT WITH NATURE** whenever possible, for a vital recharge.

AVOID

herbs that may dry up your milk supply, such as sage, peppermint, parsley leaf, spearmint and yarrow.

DAILY PROTOCOL

Postnatal Depletion

Morning and Evening	Throughout the Day
### DROP the **Mama Nourish Elixir** (p. 228) onto the tongue. This nutritive blend delivers an extra vitamin-rich and mineral-dense boost, while boosting immunity and offering the nervous system a reassuring, healthful hug. ### COOK with the **Scrap Broth** (p. 119) as a base for recipes, as a way to ultra-charge meals with nourishment. Use this broth as you would a stock for a recipe base, in soups, stews, grain-based meals, and so on.	### SIP on the **Nettle and Oat Straw Infusion** (p. 68), a radically restorative earthy combo to refuel a tank empty of vitality and resilience. Nettle leaf and oat straw are also super-helpful galactagogues, bringing the added bonus of milk-production support, if needed. ### SNACK on a few **Heroic Bliss Balls** (p. 225). These eye-opening (yet stimulant-free) treats offer a green pick-me-up that is packed full of adaptogens and nutrient-dense iron sources, paired with beneficial fats and fibre and a touch of sweetness.

Direly overlooked, postnatal depletion is an epidemic among new mothers. After growing a baby, birthing a baby and then moving on to feeding a baby – coupled with the mammoth changes that parenthood demands – it is no surprise that many women are experiencing marked postnatal depletion. This protocol is all about deep nourishment and replenishment. Follow for as long as it feels good to do so.

Enhancements

PRACTISE THE PILLARS

Bring all the Pillars to Thrive on board, with all the nourishment they provide. It is time to restore, and each of these practices will assist in recentring your body and being.

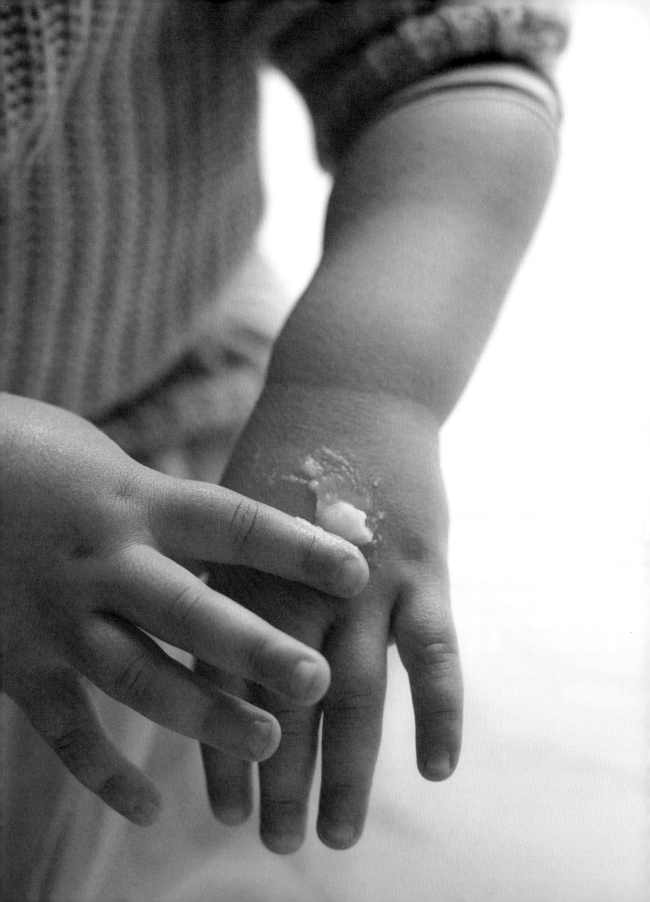

Barrier Salve

HERBAL INGREDIENTS

¼ cup dried chamomile
   flowers
¼ cup dried calendula
   flowers
¼ cup dried rosehips
¼ cup dried St John's wort
   flowers/leaf

For both little ones and grown-ups, a most helpful herbal salve to calm irritation and aggravation of the skin. With a soothing herbal-infused oil base, this nourishing blend deeply hydrates the dermal layers. This salve is wonderful for rashes of all sorts, including nappy rash, eczema and dermatitis, and for general skin dryness.

METHOD

First, make the Herbal-Infused Oil base recipe (p. 31) with the herbal ingredients.

Now, make the Salve base recipe (p. 36) using your infused oil.

DOSAGE

Keep irritated skin moist by applying frequently and liberally.

See Nappy Rash (p. 233)

MUMS AND BUBS

Calendula Tea

A simple calendula-flower tea infusion, cooled and used as a wash, can be a soothing force for treating wounds, cuts, irritations and abrasions.

HERBAL INGREDIENT

2 teaspoons dried calendula flowers

METHOD

Make the Wash base recipe (p. 39) with the calendula flowers.

See Mastitis (p. 232); Post-Birth Support (p. 232)

Calm Tum Tea

Chamomile and fennel bring a reassuring energy and usher in calm relief. This tea is deal for intestinal colic, gas build-up or digestive discomfort. Although the pleasant-on-the-palate blend is particularly fitting for little ones, it has the ability to help all in need, irrespective of age. It's generally not recommended that babies under the age of 6 months old digest herbal teas directly, however if your infant is purely breastfed, you can drink 3 cups of this tea and will absolutely see the positive impacts flow to the little one through your lactation. If your bub is formula fed, you can add 1 teaspoon of a herbal tea into a bottle of formula. If you are offering any infant a herbal tea, it is always best to cool and dilute the tea with extra cold water first.

HERBAL INGREDIENTS

2 teaspoons dried chamomile flowers
2 teaspoons dried fennel seeds

METHOD

Make the Medicinal Tea base recipe (p. 33) with the herbal ingredients.

See Colic (p. 233)

Chamomile Wash

So simple, and so soothing. Chamomile washes are lovely for skin irritations, and are particularly helpful for infants and little ones – ideal for nappy rash.

HERBAL INGREDIENT

2 teaspoons dried
    chamomile flowers

METHOD

Make the Wash base recipe (p. 39) with the chamomile flowers.

See Nappy Rash (p. 233)

Comfrey Salve

A simple saviour, this skin salve is centred around the wonderful comfrey plant. Offering topical pain relief and a cooling impact on inflammation, this all-rounder remedy has an endless number of uses. Particularly wonderful for soothing back pain, cracked skin and nipples, fractured bones and sprains, strains and muscular aches.

HERBAL INGREDIENTS

½ cup dried comfrey leaf
½ cup dried comfrey root

METHOD

First, make the Herbal-Infused Oil base recipe (p. 31) with the herbal ingredients.

Now, make the Salve base recipe (p. 36) using your infused oil.

See Cracked Nipples (p. 232)

MUMS AND BUBS

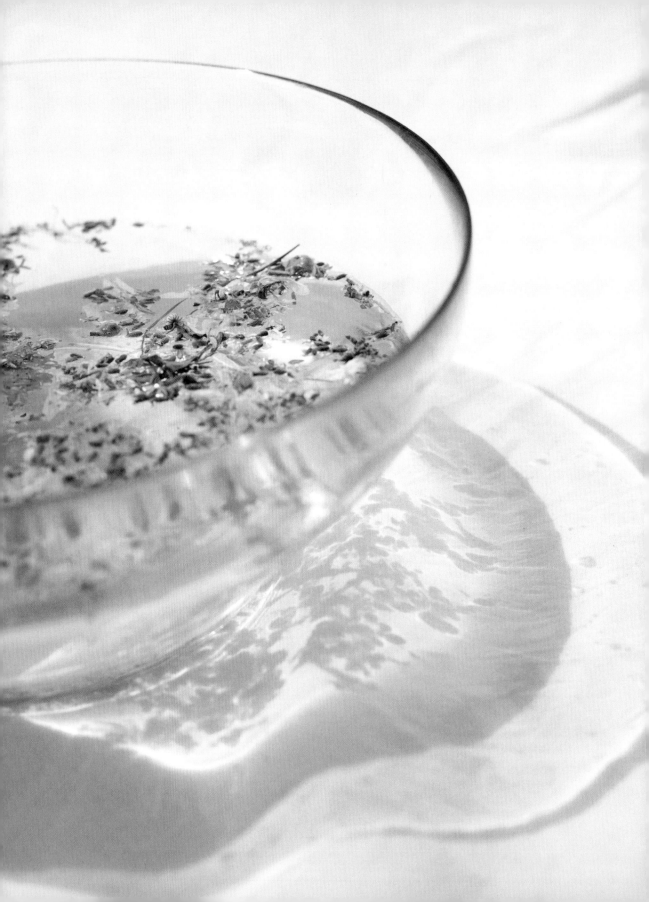

Floral Post-Birth Sitz Bath

HERBAL INGREDIENTS

1 cup Epsom salts or Dead Sea salts

3 tablespoons dried yarrow flowers/leaf

3 tablespoons dried lavender flowers

3 tablespoons dried calendula flowers

3 tablespoons dried chamomile flowers

3 tablespoons dried comfrey leaf

2 tablespoons dried marshmallow root

4 tablespoons dried witch-hazel leaf

Note: If you want to use this reparative blend in a spritz bottle to spray tissues in need or to saturate a sanitary pad (extra wonderful popped into the fridge to cool before wearing), simply brew your medicinal tea as described above, and add in ¼ cup Epsom or Dead Sea salts while the tea is infusing. Allow to cool, then decant into your spray bottle.

After giving birth, the perineal tissues often need extra TLC. This blend is perfect for a sitz bath. With a slight change in preparation, it can also be popped into a spray bottle and used to spritz areas in need or to saturate a sanitary pad, to cool inflammation and irritation. Sitz baths offer the vaginal tissues and surrounding area a super-cooling wave of healing – they have been utilised in this way for centuries. This blend is also super helpful for post C-section birth: when the tissues are past the point of acute healing, gently spritz to encourage wound healing. Angry haemorrhoids will also deeply appreciate this herbal practice.

METHOD

Make the Medicinal Tea base recipe (p. 33) with the herbal ingredients, but leave the salts out for now.

Run a warm bath. While the water is running, add the medicinal tea along with the salts.

Immerse yourself in the bath for 20 minutes to allow healing to take place.

Repeat frequently!

See Post-Birth Support (p. 232)

MUMS AND BUBS

Herbal Talc Powder

Many of us remember being covered in white clouds of talcum powder as infants, only to find out later that most of these products were full of undesirable chemicals! Here we have a clean herbal version with which to pamper our little ones. Encouraging soothing and softness, this talc is super easy to make, and can be dusted on after the bath, or used to calm nappy rash and skin irritations.

HERBAL INGREDIENTS

½ cup arrowroot

¼ cup bentonite clay

½ tablespoon lavender
   powder

1½ tablespoons calendula
   powder

1½ tablespoons
   chamomile powder

1½ tablespoons
   marshmallow powder

METHOD

Mix powders together thoroughly.

Store in an airtight sealed jar.

DOSAGE

Apply liberally on the skin, multiple times daily as needed.

See Nappy Rash (p. 233)

Heroic Bliss Balls

Laced with energy-yielding elements, super greens and adaptogenic plants, these wholesome pick-me-ups will naturally elevate your vitality. This recipe has a flexible nature, and you can swap out seeds, sweeteners and nut butters with ease – just be sure to stick to the quantity guidelines.

MAKES UP TO 16 BLISS BALLS

HERBAL INGREDIENTS

1 teaspoon ginger rhizome powder

1 teaspoon fennel seed powder

1 tablespoon maca root powder

1 tablespoon ashwagandha powder

NUTRITIONAL INGREDIENTS

6 Medjool dates

2 tablespoons blackstrap molasses or raw honey

½ cup pumpkin seeds

¾ cup peanut butter or nut butter of choice

1 cup unsweetened shredded coconut

¼ cup tahini

2 heaped tablespoons super greens (e.g. chlorella, spirulina or moringa powder)

METHOD

Pit the dates and soften by soaking them in a bowl of warm water for 10 minutes. Drain the dates, then place them in a food processor along with all the other ingredients.

Blitz on high until the mixture forms a dough.

Break off tablespoon-sized pieces of the dough and roll into balls. Keep in a sealed container in the fridge for up to 7 days. Alternatively, you can freeze them – simply allow the balls to defrost for 10 or so minutes until fully thawed, then enjoy.

See Postnatal Depletion Protocol (p. 216)

MUMS AND BUBS

Lactation Flow-Support Tea

Galactagogue herbs support breast-milk production, and this fresh lemony blend is chock full of them – making it a fitting formula to gift to a mama-to-be. Hydration is important to encourage free-flowing lactation, and drinking your galactagogue-rich plants is an essential act of support. This tea is perfect warm or iced.

HERBAL INGREDIENTS

4 teaspoons dried aniseed

2 teaspoons dried caraway seeds

2 teaspoons dried alfalfa leaf

6 teaspoons dried lemon verbena leaf

1 teaspoon dried fenugreek seeds

1 teaspoon dried blessed thistle

METHOD

Make the Medicinal Tea base recipe (p. 33) with the herbal ingredients. Brew this tea for 10 minutes to keep the bitterness at bay! Add a dollop of honey if sweetness is desired.

DOSAGE

If you are seeking to boost milk production, be sure to include 3–4 cups in your daily diet.

See Lactation Support Protocol (p. 214)

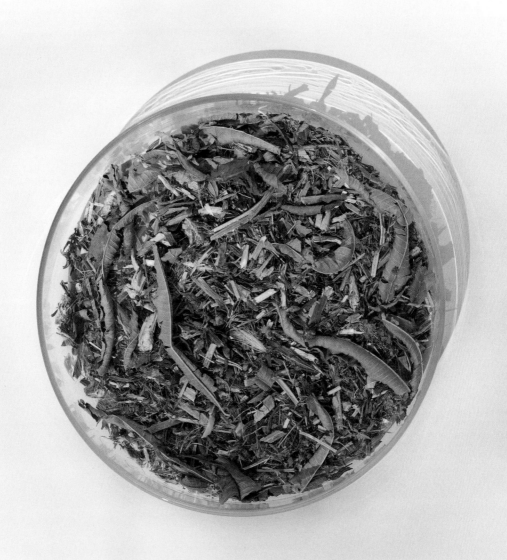

Mama Nourish Elixir

HERBAL INGREDIENTS

4 tablespoons dried
    elderberries
4 tablespoons dried oat
    straw or milky oat tops
3 tablespoons dried
    rosehips
4 tablespoons dried nettle
    leaf
2 tablespoons dried
    horsetail aerial parts
2 tablespoons dried alfalfa
    leaf
2 tablespoons dried red
    clover flowers
2 tablespoons dried
    raspberry leaf

This syrupy, herb-infused treacle is a true delight for any mama in need of a nourishing lift. Safety considerations around lactation need not prevent you bringing this plant-rich elixir on board postpartum to rebuild innate strength and fortification. Deeply nutritive and gently sweet, it is an ally for all who need it (not just mamas!).

METHOD

Make the Simple Syrup base recipe (p. 37) with the herbal ingredients.

See Lactation Support Protocol (p. 214); Postnatal Depletion Protocol (p. 216)

Milkshake Bliss Balls

NUTRITIONAL INGREDIENTS

1 cup Medjool dates

4 tablespoons almond butter or nut butter of choice

1/3 cup shredded coconut

1/3 cup whole rolled gluten-free oats

1/3 cup ground flaxseed meal

3 tablespoons gluten-free brewer's yeast

a pinch of sea salt

1/2 teaspoon vanilla powder or vanilla extract

1 heaped tablespoon of semi-soft coconut oil

Creamy, smooth, nutrient dense and super-duper easy to make: these bite-sized raw delights are a take on the traditional lactation-enhancing cookie. Harnessing key galactagogue foods, they combine oats, brewer's yeast and flaxseed meal to aid lactation support.

MAKES UP TO 16 BLISS BALLS

METHOD

Pit the dates and soften by soaking them in a bowl of warm water for 10 minutes. Drain the dates, then place them in a food processor along with all the other ingredients.

Blitz on high until the mixture forms a dough.

Break off tablespoon-sized pieces of the dough and roll into balls. Keep them in a sealed container in the fridge for up to 7 days. Alternatively, you can freeze them – simply allow the balls to defrost for 10 or so minutes, to soften, then enjoy.

DOSAGE

These make the perfect snack at any time of day for those who are breastfeeding.

See Lactation Support Protocol (p. 214)

MUMS AND BUBS

Raspberry Leaf Tea

HERBAL INGREDIENT

2 teaspoons raspberry leaf

An ultra-nourishing tisane. Raspberry leaf is a star when it comes to pregnant people, but it is not limited to that role – it supports a healthful menstrual cycle, as well as lactation, and can be taken to ease acute diarrhoea. A relative of the rose, raspberry leaf tastes quite delicious, much like black tea. It happily forms the base taste for many herbal blends, but it can also be enjoyed on its own.

METHOD

Make the Medicinal Tea base recipe (p. 33) with the raspberry leaf.

DOSAGE

Please see the information in 'For Birth Preparation and Nourishment' (p. 213) regarding consumption of raspberry leaf tea during pregnancy. It's worth noting that women are commonly advised to wait until they are 32 weeks pregnant before taking the tea.

See Fortified Pregnancy Support Protocol – For Birth Preparation and Nourishment (p. 213)

Slippery Elm Paste

HERBAL INGREDIENT

1 teaspoon dried slippery
    elm powder

Slippery elm powder is a godsend for the gut, soothing irritations such as reflux, indigestion and intestinal colic. This quick trick is mainly used to treat bubs with belly discomfort. The paste can be applied directly to the nipple when breastfeeding, or if bub has progressed to solid foods it can be mixed into puréed fruits and vegetables, or added to porridge.

METHOD

Mix the powder and 2 teaspoons water together in a small bowl until the desired consistency is achieved. You can add a little more water if you find it is too thick, or a dash more powder if it is too runny.

Spoon 1 teaspoon into mashed or puréed foods, and mix until combined. Start with lower doses to ensure bub tolerates the taste – the flavour is easier to disguise when you add these smaller amounts! Or if breastfeeding, dab some paste onto the nipples pre-feeding, for the bub to ingest when they latch on.

Offering a little extra hydration in the form of liquid or hydrating foods is a great idea when taking slippery elm, to ensure its smooth passage through the digestive tract. This is not needed in the case of breastfeeding, which delivers ample hydration.

See Colic (p. 233)
See also Dry Cough Protocol (p. 84)

MUMS AND BUBS

Rescue Remedies

For Mum

CRACKED NIPPLES

Soothe cracked, sore nipples with frequent applications of **Comfrey Salve** (p. 221) – the perfect, simple plant medicine to usher in healing. Be mindful to apply this between feeds, to avoid bub ingesting the balm!

MASTITIS

Applying cold cabbage leaves to the breast like a compress is an old folk remedy that has withstood the test of time. Be sure to ask your greengrocer for a cabbage with the large leaves intact: these are the leaves you remove to place over the breast, and they will feel extra soothing if you refrigerate them in advance. Acute-dose the **Echinacea Tincture** (p. 101) at the onset of any symptoms, and sip on cups of **Calendula Tea** (p. 220). These remedies are key in immunity support and work to clear any underlying inflammation and infection present. Rest up and stay very well hydrated. It is essential to keep feeding, or expressing breast milk, through the discomfort. I know this is much easier said than done. Vitamin C supplementation is a wonderful ally, but moderate to high doses can cause diarrhoea for bub – so definitely start at a lower dose and increase gradually. Try the **C Powder** (p. 92) added into a smoothie or stirred straight into a large glass of water.

OVERSUPPLY OF BREAST MILK

There are a few potent herbs that will absolutely work to dry up your milk supply, so please avoid them if you are not seeking this outcome! But if you do want to reduce milk supply, make a simple single-herb or combination tea with sage (see **Sage Tea**, p. 117), peppermint or yarrow leaf and sip throughout your day. For a more potent option, you could work with a single herb tincture made with just one of the above and dose on the higher side for quick impact.

POST-BIRTH SUPPORT

Plant medicines have been used for aeons to offer postnatal healing. Try the **Floral Post-Birth Sitz Bath** (p. 223), to heal the perineal tissues following a vaginal birth. This sitz bath greatly reduces swelling and inflammation, repairing tissues (if a vaginal tear is present) and improving blood flow, to provide relief and healing. It is also wonderful for haemorrhoid relief.

As a quick remedy to support tissue healing, prepare a strong **Calendula Tea** (p. 220) and mix with 1 tablespoon of aloe vera gel – this can be popped into a spray bottle and spritzed onto the vagina. Essential oils such as lavender, chamomile or tea tree are optional additions for a more aromatic experience.

PS: Homeopathic arnica will reduce swelling and bruising – an essential in any birthing kit.

For Bub

CRADLE CAP
The best way to combat this non-infectious scalp build-up is with oil. Massage a few drops of **Rosemary-Infused Olive Oil** (p. 263) onto the little one's scalp with your hands, or use a soft brush. Leave overnight and shampoo out the next day. Reapply as needed to gradually soften and clear cradle cap formation.

COLIC
Calm Tum Tea (p. 220), a simple mix of fennel seeds and chamomile flowers, will offer sweet relief for reflux or colic. **Slippery Elm Paste** (p. 231), mixed with a little breast milk and popped directly on the nipple/in a bottle, can be incredibly soothing for digestive discomfort.

PS: If the bub is breastfed, be sure to consider mum's diet, which can include foods triggering gas and discomfort. The most common offenders include spicy foods, caffeine, dairy, chocolate, soy, alcohol, gluten-containing grains, pungent foods such as garlic and onions, and gas-forming veggies such as broccoli, cauliflower and cabbage. An elimination diet can be very helpful, allowing you to check whether the absence of a certain food impacts the bub in a positive way.

NAPPY RASH
Make a simple **Chamomile Wash** (p. 221), then dip a clean, soft washcloth into the mixture, allowing it to soak up the chamomile-infused water. Gently place this on the little one's nappy rash – a quick compress of sorts, to soothe irritated skin. Pat the skin dry, dust with **Herbal Talc Powder** (p. 224) and then follow with a generous amount of **Barrier Salve** (p. 219), a soothing bum balm for bubs. Repeat this at nappy change time when possible.

TEETHING
Diluted **Chamomile Tea** (p. 161) can be very supportive for a little one experiencing the woes of cutting teeth. You can add it to a bottle or softly syringe it directly into bubba's mouth. I also suggest dipping a clean washcloth into the tea, removing and freezing it, and then offering bub the cooling cloth to chew on. Additionally, rub gentle, olive oil–based **Clove Oil** (p. 97) onto the gums, to bring a welcome sensation of numbness and relief.

MUMS AND BUBS

Hair and Skin

With unrealistic standards of beauty pounded into all of us on a daily basis, external health is an undeniably big deal. The skin is a living, breathing marvel of purpose, the ultimate reflection of your inner health universe. Beneath its surface exists an entire wonderland.

The skin creates a barrier – a human safety suit – and is part of the protective integumentary system (made up of the skin, along with hair, nails, nerves and glands), which is also heavily involved in detoxification. Skin performs a whole slew of tasks, and needs care and consideration; it is our softly set armour.

Your skin can also tell you a great deal about what is actually going on inside you. The skin, hair and nails are excellent markers of health, giving great insight into internal wellbeing. They can point to underlying issues like nutrient deficiencies; for instance, hair loss is commonly associated with low iron levels, while nail ridging is often an indicator of low calcium.

Skin is incredibly porous, so what we put on our skin matters greatly. We need to practise due diligence and become ingredient scholars when it comes to the contents of topical therapeutics and body products. Consumers, awake!

Getting to the origins of acute or chronic skin issues can be challenging, because it is, effectively, a process of elimination. Eczema is a perfect example. Although this is most definitely a skin condition, there are always other elements of health impacting or contributing to the presentation. The gut is often involved, with food intolerances and underlying digestive dysbiosis (an imbalance in gut bacteria) being linked to eczema. Emotional stress can also be a huge contributing factor, as can hormonal imbalances. But which one or which combination is the driver of a person's disruptive eczema woes?

The key is to get to the causative and contributing roots, to the heart of it all; to look at the whole, interconnected story of our external skin health, acknowledging that skin issues are not simply about what we put on our skin. What we put in our bodies can have colossal impacts on the health of our skin. We need to feed our skin: with nutrition, with water, with nature's bounty in one way or another.

The complex nature of skin health means that it is notoriously tricky to treat skin concerns, but plant medicines have a glorious dexterity when it comes to supporting the skin, the hair and the nails.

Often it is as simple as weaving in herbals to speak directly to the lymphatic system, encouraging a shift in stagnation and igniting an outer glow.

Many of the tried-and-true remedies ahead have their origins in folk medicine. These old-worldly herbal hacks speak for themselves – they have withstood the test of time! Add them to your herbal first aid kit. Try out a **Lush Locks Infusion** (p. 256) if your hair is dull, or **Rosemary-Infused Olive Oil** (p. 263) to encourage hair growth. If you have a chronic skin condition, follow these daily protocols as they lead you through the portal of skin health, and remember to look at the whole picture – nothing is one-dimensional. And, importantly, practise the Pillars to Thrive (p. 16) and honour your healing process.

Consider the following if you are struggling with skin conditions

— It is critical to look at your overall diet when you are in the process of healing skin issues. Food is absolutely your medicine. Consider the nutritional tips on page 20 to deepen your skin health and healing journey.

— Focus on drinking plenty of pure water; it's absolutely essential for skin health and clearance.

— Enjoy plenty of prebiotic- and probiotic-rich foods (see p. 20), and focus on creating a varied, wholefoods-based diet rich in antioxidant-yielding plant-based sources, such as berries, kale and broccoli. Flat out avoid (or at least reduce!) added sugar and processed foods.

— There are many nutrients that are indicated to support skin issues of all forms, but a few in particular can be very beneficial. Look to increase food sources containing the nutrients listed below, but don't be afraid to reach for supplements to up your intake if needed. Be sure to check in with a qualified practitioner for dosage guidelines and personal prescription.

Some skin nourishing superstars

— Evening primrose oil
— Fish oils
— Probiotics
— Selenium
— Vitamins A, C, D, E
— Zinc

A gentle heads up

Please do not let this deter you, but if you are working on a stubborn skin issue herbally and naturally, be aware that you may get a flare-up before it gets better. Consult your friendly herbalist, naturopath or other qualified practitioner, and persist if it feels right. Often a breakthrough is just around the corner.

Acne

Morning	Throughout the Day
POP the **Hepato-Cleanse Caps** (p. 134) with breakfast, to support the liver gently but surely.	**DRINK** **Clear Frontier Tea** (p. 248), for lymphatic support. Brew this tea super strong. **DAB** **The Breakout Salve** (p. 247) onto acne-prone areas, to minimise redness and scarring. With a castor oil and beeswax base, this herbal-infused balm acts to decongest and nurture.

Acne can be a persistent and relentless source of trouble, and it is important to isolate the triggers contributing to your breakouts. Consider hormone imbalances, food sensitivities, gut health and stress as major factors. The guided prescription below offers up many much-loved herbal skin remedies to encourage harmonic dermal healing.

Enhancements

PRACTISE THE PILLARS

HYDRATION is a major player for clear skin. Make a conscious effort to drink water. Focus on cleaning up your diet and eating really **GOOD FOOD**. If you are feeling strung-out and stressed, pave the way for **REST**. Be sure to connect with your internal **SELF-TALK**. Feeling self-conscious about your skin can be very challenging, so go gently with yourself. Get into the sun and **CONNECT WITH NATURE** – sunshine therapy is key for skin healing.

HAIR AND SKIN

DAILY PROTOCOL

DAILY PROTOCOL

Dull Skin

Morning	Throughout the Day	
BLEND yourself a **Green Dream Smoothie** (p. 131), alchemised with the **Skin Shroom Booster** (p. 265), a blended medicinal-mushroom powder of chaga, tremella and reishi, to encourage radiance.	**DRINK** **Shifting Stagnancy Tea** (p. 141), a strong, lymphatic-supporting herbal blend to aid clearance and blood cleansing, all key for shining skin. *or* **SIP** **Glowing Skin Tea** (p. 252), which by the way tastes wonderful iced.	
Enhancements	**CONSIDER** adding in the ancient Chinese healing practice of Gua Sha to enliven circulation and lymphatic flow and activate glow.	

For when you are feeling less than luminous, bring this plant-tastic protocol on to reboot your inner shine. When the skin feels dull, sallow or congested, it is a dazzling idea to employ a gentle skin cleanse full of lymphatic-loving herbs and skin-supportive practices to clear, fortify and shift stagnancy. Give this protocol a good 4 weeks to work its magic.

Afternoon	Evening
SNACK on **Incandescent Chocolates** (p. 254), highly antioxidant and dense in cacao and herbs. Although they feel decadent, they are totally therapeutic.	**SMOOTH ON** the **Manuka and Matcha Mask** (p. 259), to encourage hydrated, bright, dewy skin. **MOISTURISE** your body with **Calendula Oil** (p. 247), to encourage supple and sparkly hydrated skin. This simple oil is infused with the cheerful, sunny flowers of calendula.

PRACTISE THE PILLARS

Bring all of the Pillars on board to improve general health, and your skin will follow suit. **HYDRATE**, hydrate, hydrate: water is the skin's greatest friend! Eat **GOOD FOOD**, with a focus on plenty of plant based foods and good fats (discussed on p. 20). Be sure to sweat it out and encourage lymphatic flow with **BODY MOVEMENT**. Be mindful of **SELF-TALK** – you are beautiful. Let the sun kiss your skin: **CONNECT WITH NATURE**.

Eczema / Dermatitis

Throughout the Day	Evening
SIP	**SOAK**
Clear Frontier Tea (p. 248), a potent brew full of lymphatic-supportive herbs to stimulate the lymphatic system and clear skin concerns.	in a soothing **Oaty Bath** (p. 261). There is simply nothing better to calm irritated skin than a bath full of milky oat-infused water. Aim to do this daily when your eczema is aggravated.
APPLY	*or*
the **Eczema Cream** (p. 250), a beloved blend with a vitamin E and manuka honey base. Smooth this onto any eczema patches, rubbing it in gently, and apply whenever the skin begins to feel dry or irritated. You can also use the **All Purpose Salve** (p. 246) to keep your skin moisturised and supple.	**APPLY**
	the simple **Skin Porridge Poultice** (p. 264) on the skin as a paste. Leave for 10–20 minutes, then rinse off.

These two skin conditions often present in much the same way, and methods of treatment can be quite interchangeable. You can utilise the following skin-supportive guide to encourage a reduction in skin inflammation and irritability.

Enhancements

PRACTISE THE PILLARS

Stay well **HYDRATED**. Focus on nourishing, **GOOD FOOD** and a clean diet. Check in with your stress levels and allow yourself **REST**. Bring on daily **BODY MOVEMENT** to encourage lymphatic system flow.

CONSIDER

adding a squeeze of lemon juice and 1 teaspoon of chlorella powder to a tall glass of room-temperature water. This quick cocktail is supportive for the liver, aiding gentle detoxification and adding beneficial skin nutrition.

HAIR AND SKIN

DAILY PROTOCOL

DAILY PROTOCOL

Psoriasis

Upon Rising	Morning and Evening	
DRINK the ultra-green **Liver-Lovin' Greens Powder** (p. 136), mixed into a tall glass of room-temperature water, to aid gentle detoxification and add beneficial skin nutrition.	**POP** the **Dermal Cleanser Capsules** (p. 248), a psoriasis-specific blend to assist the liver and act as a blood cleanser, which in turn majorly impacts the skin. With Oregon grape, St Mary's thistle, burdock and bupleurum, this blend of herbal allies will work hard to shift the underlying liver, immune and lymphatic dysfunction causing the symptoms of psoriasis.	
Enhancements	**CONSIDER** working on gut healing and reducing pro-inflammatory elements in your diet and lifestyle, as psoriasis responds best to a truly holistic approach.	

Although often mistaken for eczema, psoriasis is actually an autoimmune condition characterised by an overproduction of skin cells. Acute flare-ups can occur, but generally psoriasis is a (very) chronic issue. This protocol offers insight into addressing elemental areas of the body that need extra support, as a way to control and clear psoriasis.

	Throughout the Day	Evening
	APPLY the **Eczema Cream** (p. 250) to the skin, and rub in gently. Be sure to keep the skin moist by applying the cream multiple times daily.	**SOAK** in an **Oaty Bath** (p. 261), to soothe the skin. *or* **APPLY** the quick **Skin Porridge Poultice** (p. 264).

PRACTISE THE PILLARS

HYDRATE well. Eat **GOOD FOOD**, this really is key. Address underlying stressors, and carve out **REST**. **CONNECT WITH NATURE** with sun exposure – UVB light is incredibly healing for psoriasis. So is the ocean, so if you can get to the beach, immerse yourself in seawater, stat!

HAIR AND SKIN

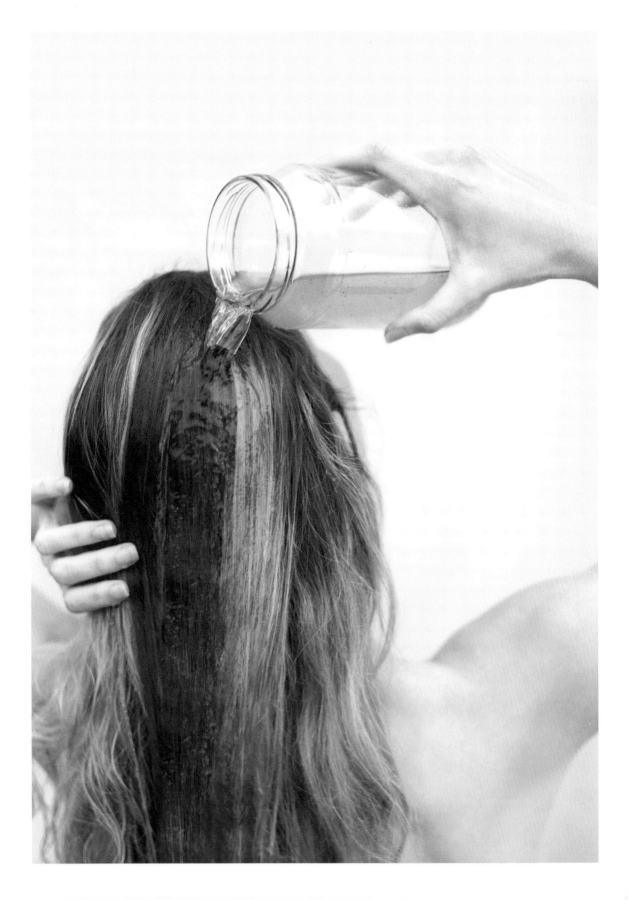

ACV Balancing Hair Rinse

Parched and overly oily scalps often produce problematic flaky dandruff – if this is an issue for you, give this herbal rinse remedy a good go. Apple cider vinegar serves as a base here, helping to course-correct dandruff build-up, calm frizz and encourage hair shine. The inclusion of scalp-loving herbals makes this a beautiful blend to rinse over clean hair to encourage a healthy scalp.

HERBAL INGREDIENTS

- ¼ cup unpasteurised apple cider vinegar
- 2 tablespoons dried rosemary
- 2 tablespoons dried nettle leaf
- 2 tablespoons dried horsetail aerial parts
- 2 tablespoons dried oat straw

METHOD

Make the Medicinal Tea base recipe (p. 33) with the herbal ingredients to create a strong infused tea. Once it is well brewed, allow to cool to lukewarm, then add the apple cider vinegar. And pour!

DOSAGE

This rinse is most effective if used after every hair wash throughout your week and can be left in to dry.

See Dandruff (p. 268)

HAIR AND SKIN

All-Purpose Salve

HERBAL INGREDIENTS

¼ cup dried calendula
   flowers
¼ cup dried chickweed
   aerial parts
¼ cup dried marshmallow
   root
¼ cup dried comfrey leaf/
   root

Hail the heal-all herbal salve! A seriously handy salve to have in any home, it is perfect for rashes, itchy bites, and dry and irritated skin. It is also a beloved boo-boo salve for any little one learning to be in the world, with all the bumps and scrapes that this entails. I consider this an essential for any home gardener who is weathering scratches and sore hands.

METHOD

First, make the Herbal-Infused Oil base recipe (p. 31) with the herbal ingredients.

Now, make the Salve base recipe (p. 36) using your infused oil.

See Eczema/Dermatitis (p. 240)
See also Rashes (p. 301); Stings and Bites (p. 302)

Antiviral Tincture

HERBAL INGREDIENTS

½ cup dried St John's wort
   flowers/leaf
½ cup dried echinacea
   root/leaf/flowers
½ cup dried lemon balm
   leaf
¼ cup dried burdock root

Quell shingles and herpes breakouts with this antiviral-rich tinctured formula. At the onset of any symptoms, however mild, bring this blend on board – it a good idea to have some pre-prepared tincture sitting snugly in your herbal first aid cabinet at all times, to be called upon when needed. Echinacea and burdock work with antiviral St John's wort and lemon balm to support immunity and clear herpes viral manifestations.

METHOD

Make the Tincture base recipe (p. 38) with the herbal ingredients.

DOSAGE

Dose frequently and acutely at the onset of symptoms, following the dosing guidelines (p. 45).

See Shingles (p. 268)
See also Chickenpox (p. 122)

The Breakout Salve

HERBAL INGREDIENTS

¼ cup dried white willow bark

¼ cup dried yarrow leaf/ flowers

¼ cup dried lavender leaf

¼ cup dried comfrey leaf

20 drops tea tree essential oil

2 tablespoons castor oil

Stringent, cooling and reparative herbs join forces in this topical salve, to combat reactive skin and soothe breakouts. White willow bark – rich in the active component salicin, a common derivative ingredient in many skin-care products – has been added for its anti-inflammatory and antibacterial properties. This salve is suitable for quelling angry blemishes and assists in the healing of acne-prone areas, where scarring is a common issue.

METHOD

First, make the Herbal-Infused Oil base recipe (p. 31) with the herbal ingredients.

Now, make the Salve base recipe (p. 36) using your infused oil. Use just ¾ of a cup of your herbal-infused oil and add 2 tablespoons of castor oil alongside the beeswax. This forms a more breakout-friendly base for the salve!

DOSAGE

Gently dab onto the area in need, and apply regularly.

See Acne Protocol (p. 236)

Calendula Oil

HERBAL INGREDIENT

1 cup dried calendula flowers

An essential herbal oil to have in your home apothecary! Delightfully nourishing rubbed into the body on its own or blended into salves, forming the base for many wonderful plant-rich skin products.

METHOD

Make the Herbal-Infused Oil base recipe (p. 31) with the calendula flowers.

See Dull Skin Protocol (p. 238)

HAIR AND SKIN

Clear Frontier Tea

HERBAL INGREDIENTS

1 ½ teaspoons dried
   burdock root
2 teaspoons dried cleavers
   stem/leaf/seeds
3 teaspoons dried red
   clover flowers
2 teaspoons dried
   echinacea root/leaf/
   flowers

A loaded lymphatic blend to aid congested skin woes – ideal for inflammatory skin conditions such as eczema. Lymphatic herbs work to purify and cleanse the blood, assisting congested fluids to drain away from inflammatory sites while also providing essential nutrients so that lymphatic fluids can work their tissue-repair magic. Consider burdock, cleavers, red clover and echinacea your trusty allies, and please be patient with your process when working with skin issues – these things truly do take time.

METHOD

Make the Medicinal Tea base recipe (p. 33) with the herbal ingredients.

See Acne Protocol (p. 236); Eczema/Dermatitis Protocol (p. 240)

Dermal Cleanser Capsules

HERBAL INGREDIENTS

½ tablespoon Oregon
   grape root/bark powder
1 tablespoon St Mary's
   thistle seed powder
1 tablespoon burdock root
   powder
½ tablespoon bupleurum
   root powder

An encapsulated liver-loving meets skin-supportive formula, specific for flare-ups or chronic psoriasis, although absolutely not limited to this – you should consider these caps for any condition where the liver, immune system or lymphatic system are impacted. Capsules really aid compliance with this blend, which can be hard to stomach when taken in a powdered form!

METHOD

Make the Capsules base recipe (p. 29) with the herbal ingredients.

DOSAGE

Psoriasis is generally a chronic issue. If this is the case, follow the chronic dose advice given in the dosing guidelines (p. 44) and allow the plants time to take effect.

See Psoriasis Protocol (p. 242)

Fungal Foot Soak

Totally common and totally troublesome! Fungal nail issues can be incredibly persistent and are challenging to shift, so give this easy-to-prep foot soak a solid go. Antimicrobial herbs mixed with potent essential oils work to shift fungal formation and prevent new growth.

HERBAL INGREDIENTS

¼ cup unpasteurised
  apple cider vinegar
2 teaspoons dried lavender
  flowers
2 tablespoons dried
  eucalyptus leaf or
  5 drops eucalyptus
  essential oil
2 tablespoons dried
  thyme or 5 drops thyme
  essential oil
5 drops tea tree essential
  oil

METHOD

Add the herbal ingredients to a large round basin or bucket. Fill the basin with warm water.

Submerge your feet in the infused herbal water and soak for 10–15 minutes. You can supercharge this practice with a relaxing meditation or by listening to soothing music.

Dry your feet thoroughly and gently, drain your foot-bath water and compost your spent bath herbs.

DOSAGE

Bear in mind, this practice yields best results when implemented every night for 6 or more weeks.

See Fungal Nails/Athlete's Foot (p. 268)

HAIR AND SKIN

Eczema Cream

Note: Please be mindful that
if you use alcohol-based
tinctures you should never
apply them to cracked, open
skin – it will sting like hell, to put
it bluntly!

Tip: To give these creams a
super whippy consistency
whizz all combined ingredients
with an immersion blender.

Eczema often presents with extreme dryness, redness, itchiness
and mad irritation. Try this herbal remedy – it is my all-time
favourite go-to eczema cream formula, which I have been using
for years in my clinic! There are two ways to make this blend:
with tinctured herbs or with powdered herbs. The powdered
herbs will yield a slightly grittier cream, which is nevertheless
soothing and totally effective. The addition of manuka honey
makes a huge difference in this blend, and aids speedy healing
and tissue recovery.

HERBAL INGREDIENTS: TINCTURE FORMULA

3 tablespoons dried chamomile flowers
3 tablespoons dried licorice root
3 tablespoons dried gotu kola leaf
3 tablespoons calendula flowers
ready-made vitamin E cream
1 tablespoon aloe vera juice or fresh aloe vera plant inner gel
2 tablespoons high-grade manuka honey (if unavailable, use
   unpasteurised raw honey)

METHOD

Make the Tincture base recipe (p. 38) using the dried
chamomile flowers, licorice root, gotu kola leaf and
calendula flowers. In a sterilised bowl add 3 tablespoons
of the completed tincture formula to 4–6 tablespoons of
ready-made vitamin E cream, then stir in the aloe vera juice
and honey until well combined – all the liquid should be
absorbed by the mix. If it is a touch on the runny side, add a
little more cream to achieve the desired consistency.

Keep this cream in the fridge at all times, to extend its shelf
life to between 2 and 4 months.

HERBAL INGREDIENTS: POWDER FORMULA

1 tablespoon chamomile powder

1 tablespoon licorice powder

1 tablespoon gotu kola powder

1 tablespoon calendula powder

ready-made vitamin E cream

1 tablespoon aloe vera powder

2 tablespoons high-grade manuka honey (if unavailable, use
   unpasteurised raw honey)

METHOD

This recipe is super easy to make. In a sterilised bowl,
simply add your herbal ingredients to 4–6 tablespoons of
ready-made vitamin E cream and mix until well combined.

Keep this cream in the fridge at all times, to extend its shelf
life to between 1 and 2 months.

DOSAGE : BOTH FORMULAS

Apply frequently if eczema is present. Do your best to keep
skin moistened with the cream at all times, to avoid dryness.

See Eczema/Dermatitis Protocol (p. 240); Psoriasis Protocol (p. 242)

Glowing Skin Tea

A fresh-vibed delight for the skin, this fruity blend offers a wealth of support, encouraging dull skin to regain shine. Vitamin C–rich rosehip and lime peel offer their antioxidant powers, creating layered, zingy base notes. Sip iced, in the sunshine.

HERBAL INGREDIENTS

1 teaspoon dried alfalfa leaf

3 teaspoons dried rosehips

3 teaspoons dried passionflower leaf

2 teaspoons dried lime peel or 4 teaspoons fresh lime peel

1 teaspoon dried calendula flowers

METHOD

Make the Medicinal Tea base recipe (p. 33) or Overnight Water Infusion base recipe (p. 34) with the herbal ingredients.

See Dull Skin Protocol (p. 238)

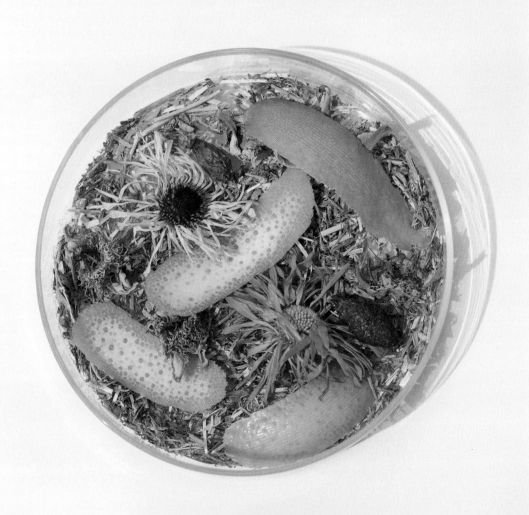

Incandescent Chocolates

HERBAL INGREDIENTS

3 tablespoons tremella powder
1 ½ tablespoons schisandra berry powder
1 teaspoon reishi powder
2 teaspoons cinnamon powder

NUTRITIONAL INGREDIENTS

a pinch of sea salt
½ cup raw cacao powder
½ cup cacao butter
½ cup coconut oil
3 tablespoons maple syrup
½ teaspoon vanilla powder or vanilla extract

Skin-loving schisandra berry, reishi, warming cinnamon and malty tremella mushroom transform these chocolate delights into a medicinal bite. Blended with the 'food of the gods' – the velvety, sacred cacao plant – and sweetened with syrup from the mighty maple tree, these plant-rich gems make the perfect afternoon pick-me-up to ignite a little luscious buzz within.

MAKES UP TO 12 CHOCOLATES

METHOD

Place the sea salt, tremella, schisandra, reishi, cinnamon and cacao powder in a clean glass bowl and mix until well combined.

In a saucepan, gently melt the cacao butter and coconut oil and then add it to the dry ingredients, along with the maple syrup and vanilla. Mix with a wooden spoon until well combined.

Pour the mixture into silicon candy or chocolate moulds. Or pour into a 20 x 20–centimetre (8 x 8 inch) brownie pan lined with baking paper, for a no-fuss chocolate bark!

Place in the fridge to set for at least 2 hours. Gently pop the chocolates out of the moulds, or break the bark into rustic pieces, and enjoy.

See Dull Skin Protocol (p. 238)

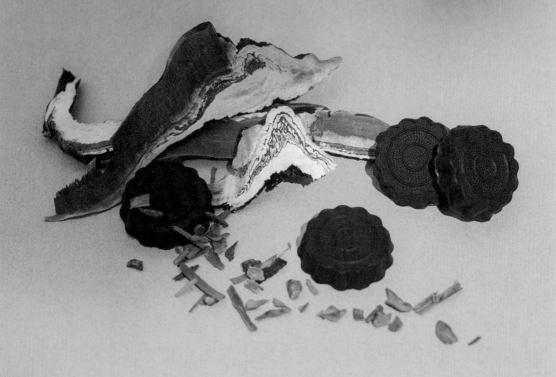

Lush Locks Infusion

HERBAL INGREDIENTS

3 tablespoons dried nettle
　leaf
1 tablespoon dried hibiscus
　flower
3 tablespoons dried
　horsetail aerial parts

Accelerate hair and nail growth with the help of this deeply brewed infusion. Nettle, hibiscus and horsetail join forces to encourage stimulation of hair follicles with their mineral-rich, collagen-emboldening properties. Make this a regular practice if you are actively seeking to strengthen and spur-on lush locks and nails.

METHOD

Make the Overnight Water Infusion base recipe (p. 34) with the herbal ingredients. Be sure to slow-brew this blend overnight!

See Poor Hair Growth (p. 268); Strong Nails (p. 268)

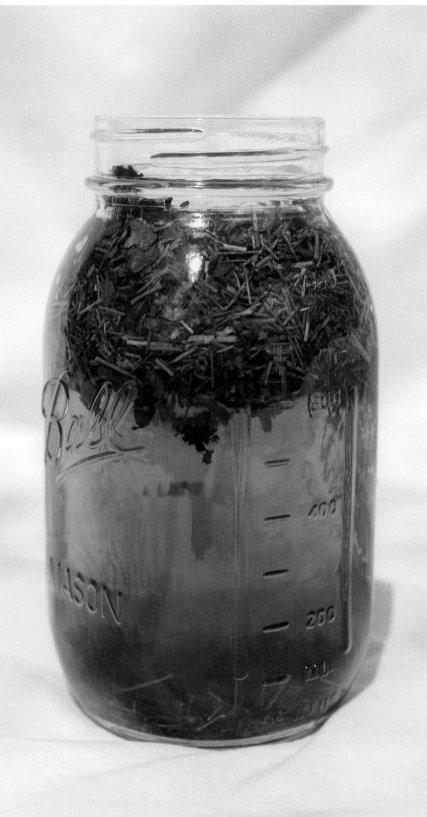

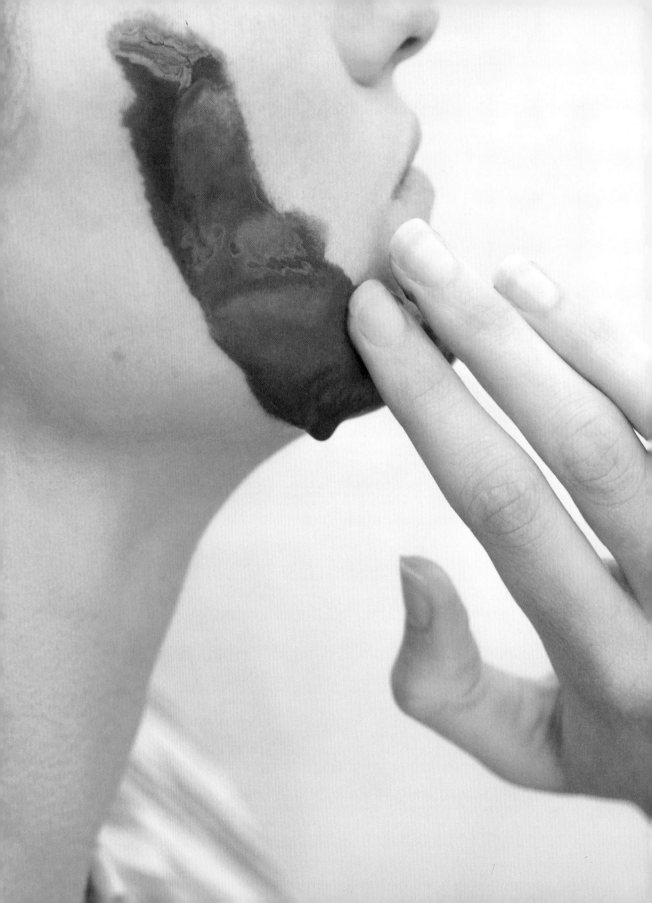

Manuka and Matcha Mask

HERBAL INGREDIENTS

1 teaspoon matcha powder
1 tablespoon manuka
  honey

Radiant skin comes from within, but feeding the skin topically is also key to bolstering luminosity. Antioxidant-rich matcha contains epigallocatechin gallate (EGCG), which works to prime skin elasticity and adjust uneven skin tones, perfect for addressing inflamed or reactive breakouts. Stellar, enzyme-rich manuka honey brings anti-inflammatory, antibacterial, antioxidant and many other beneficial anti actions! A very simple, accessible practice, to ignite a little glow.

METHOD

Mix the matcha and manuka honey in a clean small bowl until well combined.

Apply to freshly cleansed skin. Simply dip clean fingers into the brilliant green paste, and with gentle strokes cover the skin completely, avoiding the eye areas and the mouth.

Leave on the skin for 20 minutes and wash off with a compress, saturated in warm water.

DOSAGE

This mask is great to apply weekly or twice weekly to deeply nurture the skin.

See Dull Skin Protocol (p. 238)

HAIR AND SKIN

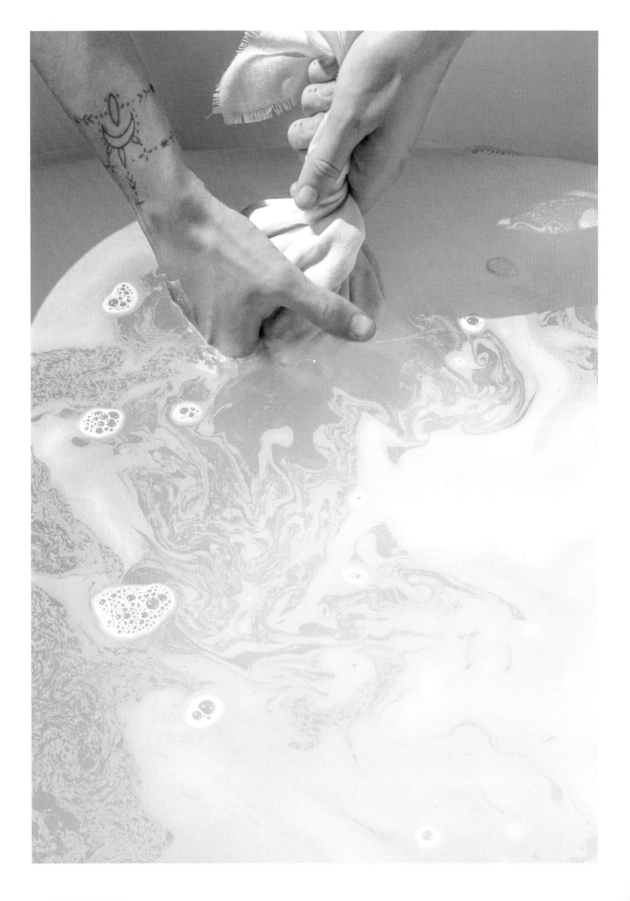

Oaty Bath

HERBAL INGREDIENT

1 cup whole rolled oats

Many of us have childhood memories of the milky waters of an oat bath. This beyond-basic kitchen remedy offers a world of soothing relief for itchy, dry, irritated skin. Perfect for eczema and dermatitis, chickenpox and seasonal skin dryness.

METHOD

You can either put the oats in a blender and pulse to create a finer meal, or pop the oats into a nut mylk bag or stocking.

Run a warm bath – be sure to avoid a very hot bath, as this can be irritating for the skin.

If you chose the blended option, pour the ground oats directly into the bath while the water is running. Alternatively, put the oat-stuffed bag/stocking in the running water. The oats will infuse their milky magic.

Hop into the bath and soak for 20 minutes, gently rubbing your body with the oat-infused water.

Once you have finished your bath, you can rinse off your skin if there are any excess oats lingering – although ideally you should just pat yourself dry!

Repeat 2–4 times weekly when the skin is irritated.

See Eczema/Dermatitis Protocol (p. 240); Psoriasis Protocol (p. 242)
See also Chickenpox (p. 122); Dry, Itchy Skin (p. 268)

HAIR AND SKIN

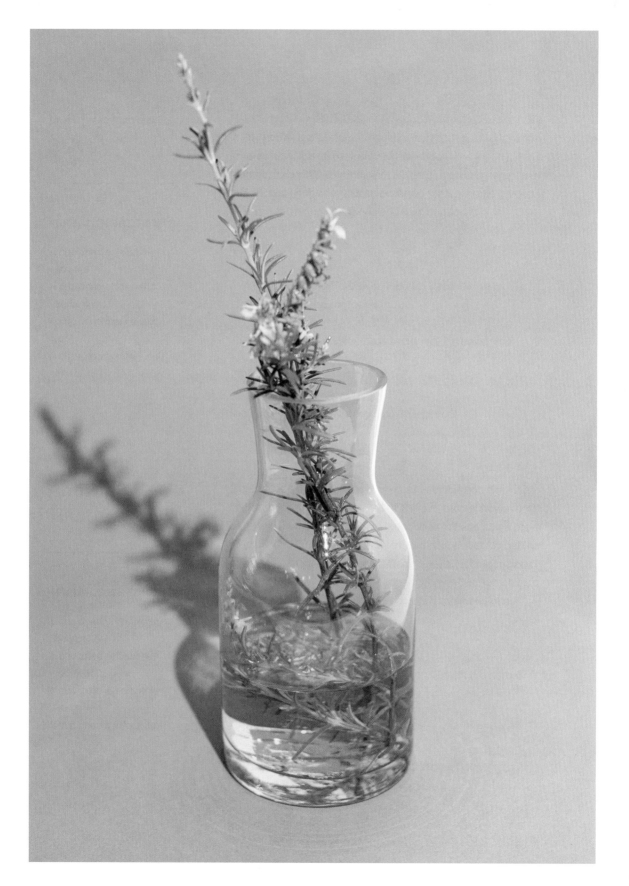

Rosemary-Infused Olive Oil

HERBAL INGREDIENT

1 cup coarsely chopped dried rosemary or 2 cups coarsely chopped fresh rosemary sprigs/leaf/flowers

A kindred pair, rosemary and olive oil meet to create a fragrant infusion that is equally edible and medicinal. A little-known application for this blend is as an aid to hair growth! If this is something you are seeking, make it a regular practice to rub this infused oil into your scalp before bed and rinse/wash out the next day. Yes, the oil can tarnish your pillowcases, but your accelerated hair growth makes it all worthwhile. This fragrant oil is also wonderful to ease cradle cap in little ones.

METHOD

Make the Herbal-Infused Oil base recipe (p. 31) with the rosemary. Be sure to use olive oil as the base oil.

Simply rub 1–2 teaspoons into the scalp multiple times weekly, leave overnight, and rinse or wash out as needed.

Be persistent with this practice and you will generally notice a marked shift after a few months of use!

See Poor Hair Growth (p. 268)
See also Cradle Cap (p. 233)

HAIR AND SKIN

Skin Porridge Poultice

This recipe is as simple as it sounds. Dollop and smooth a spoonful of oaty porridge onto irritated skin for relief from itches and irritations. *Avena sativa*, the glorious common oat, offers a wealth of demulcent healing for skin conditions of a red, dry and inflamed nature.

HERBAL INGREDIENT

¼ cup whole rolled oats

METHOD

To make a thick porridge, mix the oats and ½ cup water in a small saucepan. Bring to a boil and cook until softened, stirring frequently. Allow to cool, then follow the Poultice base recipe (p. 36).

DOSAGE

If the skin concern is acute, keep this poultice on for a good 30 minutes and reapply throughout your day.

See Eczema/Dermatitis Protocol (p. 240); Psoriasis Protocol (p. 242)

Skin Shroom Booster

HERBAL INGREDIENTS

½ teaspoon chaga powder
1 teaspoon tremella
  powder
½ teaspoon reishi powder

A trinity of tonifying medicinal mushrooms unite to nourish and enhance skin health, boosting hydration and antioxidants, and catalysing collagen production. The royals of the fungi underworld, king chaga and queen reishi, are paired with creamy and dreamy, skin-loving tremella to offer skin-supportive elements, haloed with the positive side effect of notable longevity! An easy way to include this blend in your daily rituals is to lace your favorite smoothie or plant mylk tonic with a generous dose of this shroom-dense goodness.

METHOD

Make the Herbal Powder base recipe (p. 33) with the herbal ingredients.

See Dull Skin Protocol (p. 238)

HAIR AND SKIN

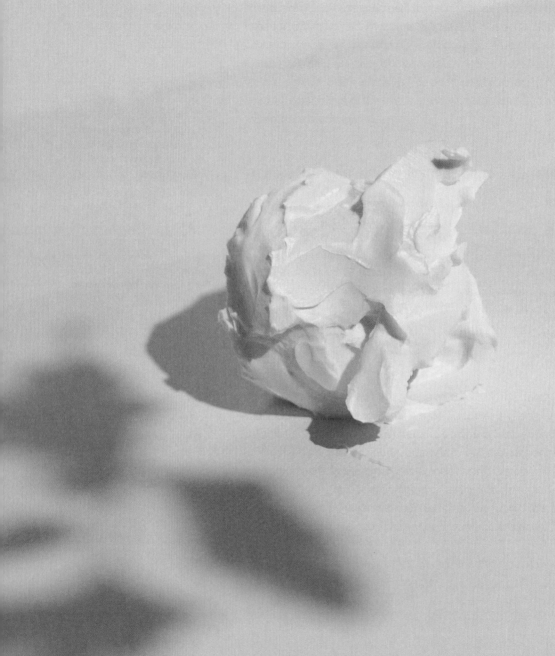

Whippy Body Butter

MAKES 2 CUPS

HERBAL INGREDIENTS

2 tablespoons dried
chamomile flowers
2 tablespoons dried
calendula flowers
2 tablespoons dried oat
straw or milky oat tops
2 tablespoons dried
rosehips
½ cup coconut oil
½ cup extra virgin olive oil
1 cup shea butter
1 teaspoon vitamin E oil
(optional)
essential oils (optional)

Dehydrated, dry, itchy and irritated skin will love you when you lather this lush butter onto your bodacious body. Body butters are intensely rich, making this recipe the perfect body moisturiser for use in cooler weather – to combat winter skin, apply a small amount to plump-up skin on the daily. A little goes a long way.

METHOD

Put your dried herbal ingredients, along with the coconut oil and olive oil, into a double boiler. Bring to a boil, reduce the heat to low and simmer for 1 hour to deeply infuse the oils with the plant material. Check regularly to make sure there is enough water in the base of the double boiler, and top up as needed. If you don't have a double boiler, place your ingredients in a heat-proof glass bowl over a saucepan filled half-full with boiling water and set to simmer as above.

Strain the herbs out with a fine-mesh sieve (and compost your spent herbs). Wipe out the double boiler and pour the strained liquid back into it. Add the shea butter to the liquid mix and stir gently until melted through.

Pour the liquid mixture into a heat- and cold-proof glass bowl and pop into the freezer for 15 minutes.

Remove from the freezer and blend the mixture with a handheld kitchen mixer on high, until completely smooth. If desired, add in your vitamin E oil and optional essential oils, and blend until combined.

Spoon into a sterilised glass jar with an airtight lid. Label, noting the ingredients, the recipe name and the date.

Store in a cool, dark cupboard. Keep in the fridge if you live in a warmer climate. This butter will stay fresh for 3 months.

See Dry, Itchy Skin (p. 268)

HAIR AND SKIN

Rescue Remedies

DANDRUFF

Cleanse your hair with **ACV Balancing Hair Rinse** (p. 245). With an apple cider vinegar base, and potentised by a long brew cycle, this herbal rinse works to correct and bring nourishment to dry, flaky imbalances of the scalp.

DRY, ITCHY SKIN

To bring moisture to dry and irritated skin, lather your awesome body generously with the **Whippy Body Butter** (p. 267), made with calendula, oat straw and chamomile, all infused in a rich oil base. This is a seriously soothing reprieve for the skin. Also be sure to immerse yourself in the demulcent arms of an **Oaty Bath** (p. 261) multiple times weekly, to butter up the skin and reduce irritation.

FUNGAL NAILS/ATHLETE'S FOOT

Persistent fungal nail issues can be the absolute pits. Many plant medicines have incredibly strong antibacterial and antimicrobial constituents and actions; in this case, bring on the **Fungal Foot Soak** (p. 249) With an apple cider vinegar base, and rich in antifungal herbals, this blend aims to clear fungal infections and keep them at bay. You must be persistent and consistent with this protocol. Follow for 6 or more weeks in order to see results.

SHINGLES

Painful and immensely uncomfortable, shingles may seem like an uncommon complaint – but, truly, they are not an anomaly at all. When stress is high, the contagious varicella-zoster virus can kick in, causing incredible neuralgic pain and blistered skin. The following suggestions work best at the very early stages of shingles onset. Follow until the shingles clear, which generally takes 7–14 days. At the very first signs of skin irritation and blister formation, apply **SJW Oil** (p. 121) topically on the skin, throughout the day. Keep this up, consistently applying every 4 hours from morning to evening. Drop a dose of the **Antiviral Tincture** (p. 246), a blended formula of St John's wort, echinacea, burdock and lemon balm, aimed at clearing the acute virus and providing swift pain relief. Follow acute dosing guidelines for best results. Be sure to stay well hydrated, to facilitate a speedier recovery. Eat good food, such as the **Scrap Broth** (p. 119), to aid immunity. Boost your beverages with the herbal **C Powder** (p. 92), to add immune-focused power. Rest is incredibly important in clearing an active virus. Consider boosting immunity with added supplementation, in the form of vitamin C, zinc and L-lysine. This trio aids in inhibiting the virus and enhances immunity.

STRONG NAILS

Drink the **Lush Locks Infusion** (p. 256) on the daily, to soak up the vitamin- and mineral-dense goodness this combo has to offer.

POOR HAIR GROWTH

Make the simply blended **Rosemary-Infused Olive Oil** (p. 263). Twice a week, rub the oil into your scalp, leave overnight and shampoo out in the morning to encourage hair growth. Drink 4 cups of mineral-rich **Lush Locks Infusion** (p. 256) daily. Made with nettles, horsetail and hibiscus, this brewed infusion supercharges hair strength, shine and growth.

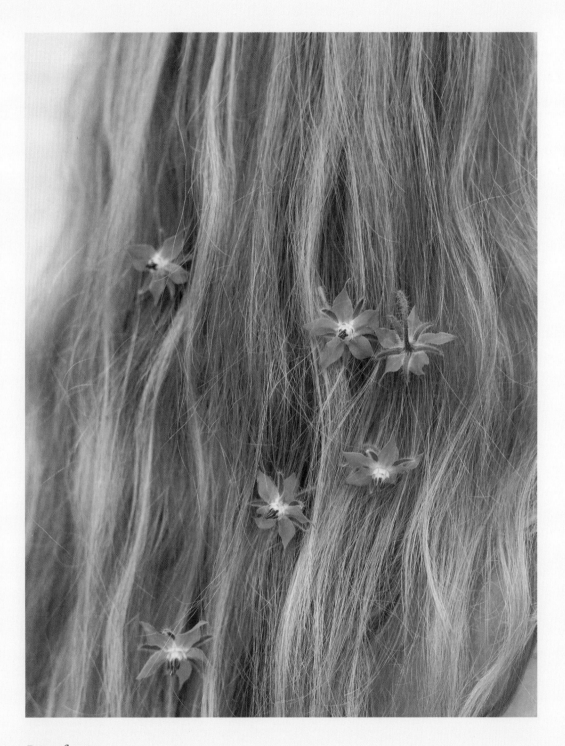

Borage flowers

Emotions, Mind, Spirit

Each of us is an ever-changing force, with our individual mood, mind state and emotional health in constant flux – at times akin to a calm forest, at other moments more like an oceanic storm, a sweeping sun-drenched plain, a barren desert, or an incandescent field of swaying flowers. We walk through many landscapes within ourselves, on a daily basis. Just like a wave, as each intangible state of being rolls in, it morphs, it passes.

Viewing plant medicines as being impactful only on the physical body is, in all honesty, a limitation. In the same way that every one of us possesses the sacred structures of the tangible body and the intangible inner workings of the mind and spirit, nature holds her own unseeable, subtle anatomies.

When you work with medicinal plants, they can be felt on many levels. Let's say, for instance, that you are feeling very anxious, perhaps a little out of body, ungrounded; your heart rate is speedy and you are feeling super overwhelmed. You drink a cup of **Calm Nerves Tea** (p. 280) and you begin to feel more grounded in your body, your heart rate eases, and the waves of overstimulation and panic subside. This transformation is felt in the body in many ways: physically, emotionally and mentally. The nervous system shifts out of the sympathetic mode (fight/flight) and glides into the parasympathetic (rest/digest) state.

Plants have a phenomenal ability to adapt their medicinal offerings to the needs of the people. They hold space for our process, bringing ease and comfort, lifting the proverbial storm clouds within us, calming the nervous system and assuring us with a warm embrace.

There is so much stigma around emotional and mental health issues. Embark on your path to healing by demystifying these spaces within yourself. From a holistic standpoint, there are many plant-centric methods and supportive elements in the pages to come that you can bring on board to usher in profound changes.

There are certain plant medicines that hold an incredible ability to speak to the emotions, the mind and the spirit. Nervines and adaptogens are two groups of plant-powered healers that truly shine in this space. From St John's wort – the sunshine chalice indicated in depression and anxiety – to hawthorn and all things rose for matters of the heart, nature has conjured up a garden of support for you and yours.

Consider these to help bring you back into balance

— Nurturing your body with nourishing food (see p. 20) will help you regulate the nervous system through nutrition and seriously support your emotional and mental wellbeing.

— Bring on some lifestyle changes! Edit out whatever does not serve you, ranging from shows or movies you may be watching to relationships that are negatively impacting your wellbeing.

— Daily body movement is so important to encourage a healthy mind and heart.

— When woven into your day, mindfulness practices, such as meditation and breathwork, are game changers. If you are overwhelmed by the thought of sitting with yourself in silence, you could do a walking meditation outside or a moving meditation like gentle yoga.

— Nature is the greatest teacher of calm and upliftment. Sit with her, be with her, soak her up.

— Talk it out. Seek a therapist or a beloved confidant who will hold space for you and your process and bring nothing but love to the situation.

Emotional states and their herbal helpers

Anger and rage
— Lavender
— Lemon balm
— Passionflower

Discouraged and without hope
— Calendula
— Saffron
— St John's wort

Exhaustion and fatigue
— Ashwagandha
— Rhodiola
— Siberian ginseng

Grief and sadness
— Hawthorn
— Motherwort
— Rose

Overstimulated
— Brahmi
— Chamomile
— Skullcap

Undernourished in body and being
— Burdock
— Nettle
— Oat straw

EMOTIONS, MIND, SPIRIT

DAILY PROTOCOL

Anxiety

Morning, Afternoon and Evening	Throughout the Day
DROP a dose of the **Peace Within Glycetract** (p. 290), a calming and grounding blend with ashwagandha, chamomile, linden and more to soothe anxiety and reshape the innate stress response. This can be taken throughout the day if anxiety is ever-present, or dosed as needed for relief and support.	SIP either the **Untangle Tea** (p. 291) or the **Calm Nerves Tea** (p. 280). Both are specifically formulated to ease anxiety and encourage a calm nervous system. EAT **Calm Candies** (p. 278), infused with passionflower, lemon balm, chamomile, skullcap and rose. Keep these candies on hand, both at home and when you are out and about; they can be a helpful on-the-go ally if you are experiencing waves of anxiety. I like to add the beloved Bach flower essence 'Rescue Remedy' to this recipe, to bring on extra calming forces.

Feeling speedy, out of body, ungrounded and hyper alert is not a comfortable experience. Luckily for us all, there is an abundance of plant medicines intrinsically primed to calm your body and being. Give this protocol a go when you are feeling anxious or experiencing stressful times. Calm body, calm mind, calm spirit.

Enhancements

PRACTISE THE PILLARS

HYDRATE to ground your body. Eat really **GOOD FOOD,** focusing on earthing and sustaining meals. Allow your body and being to **REST**. Include **BODY MOVEMENT** – lean into gentle practices like a walk out in nature. **CONNECT WITH NATURE,** even in the smallest way, for a brief period of time. Breathe and be in presence. Be mindful of your **SELF-TALK**. Visualise a tree, rooted in the earth, unshakeable and steady: you are the tree!

CONSIDER

supplementation as a super-helpful support in calming anxiety. The star minerals indicated are magnesium and calcium. A combined magnesium/calcium supplement will be a nourishing aid, while a simple magnesium, I believe, is almost essential.

DAILY PROTOCOL

Depression

Morning	Throughout the Day	
DROP the **Uplifting Oxymel** (p. 205) straight onto the tongue, or into some sparkling water for a refreshing spritzer. Made with St John's wort, borage, rosemary, rose and tulsi, this blend offers a luminescent mood-lifting bouquet. Feel free to take this multiple times per day if it feels good.	**DRINK** a cup of **Calm Nerves Tea** (p. 280), to nourish and soothe the senses and encourage an evening-out of the sympathetic nervous system (fight/flight response). **EAT** antidepressive plants where possible. Find ways to include turmeric and saffron in your cooking.	
Enhancements	**CONSIDER** weaving in key supplementation: a great B complex, magnesium, and quality omega-3 fatty acids such as fish oil, which is high in EPA and DHA. Also consider taking an encapsulated form of St John's wort. This heavily researched ray-of-sunshine herb has been praised for its ability to support and ease depression and anxiety.	

When the clouds loom and you cannot see the promise of a brighter day, the low, heavy feeling of depression can stop you in your tracks. Although it can be challenging to find motivation when you are experiencing the dark gloom of depression, give these suggestions a go. I find a solid 6 weeks of protocol compliance are needed for some of these plant medicines to work their therapy.

	Afternoon	Evening
	SNACK on a **Maca Bliss Ball** (p. 67), or two! Maca root offers mood-enhancing and inherently antidepressant properties. This recipe also aims to regulate and support your energy, offering a gentle lift.	**SOAK** in a bathtub with the **Floral Bath** (p. 281). The combination of relaxation and the sensory therapy of water and flowers dancing around you can be incredibly healing. **MASSAGE** the **Heart of Gold Salve** (p. 281) onto your body, lovingly, with particular attention given to the heart and chest area.

PRACTISE THE PILLARS

HYDRATION is uplifting for the body. Drink up! **GOOD FOOD** will be your medicine. Your body is a temple – nourish it aplenty. When you feel the need to **REST**, honour that need. Include daily **BODY MOVEMENT**, the ultimate mood lifter. Listen to your **SELF-TALK**. Be gentle on yourself. **CONNECT WITH NATURE**, soak up her therapy.

EMOTIONS, MIND, SPIRIT

Poor Focus / Cognition

Throughout the Day	Afternoon
SIP **Memory Tea** (p. 290), made with key neuro-enhancing herbs. These include brahmi, ginkgo and gotu kola – plants hailed for their power to ignite mental clarity and sharpness. **DOSE UP** on the **Timelessness Tincture** (p. 73), with a medley of cognition-supportive herbals to illuminate and hone neurological focus.	**DRINK** the **Lion's Mane Tonic** (p. 286). This milky elixir harnesses the forces of the esteemed lion's mane, transforming the medicinal 'mind mushroom' into a delicious afternoon delight to assist any 3 pm brain slumps. *or* **EAT** 1–2 **Maca Bliss Balls** (p. 67) for an energy-dense, brain-loving treat! Filled with beneficial omega 3–rich goodies, such as walnuts, hemp seeds and chia seeds, these delicious bites pack a mighty supportive punch.

Many of us often find our focus waning throughout the day. With so many wonderful cognition-enhancing plant medicines available to home apothecaries, we can lean on their supportive bounty to sharpen the mind and reignite cerebral power.

Enhancements

PRACTISE THE PILLARS

HYDRATION combats a fuzzy mind, water is focus therapy at it's very best! Fuel your body with **GOOD FOOD**, this is so essential to thrive and sustain a sharp mind. When you feel unfocused, allow yourself to **REST**. Add in a little **BODY MOVEMENT** and take yourself on a walk, shake out your body. Even better, when you take that walk **CONNECT TO NATURE** by heading outside, taking some deep breaths and resetting your ability to return to the task at hand.

CONSIDER

increasing the amount of omega-3 fatty acids in your diet (such as wild-caught fish, walnuts and chia seeds) and/or supplementation (such as a great-quality fish oil). EPA and DHA are wonderful for the brain.

EMOTIONS, MIND, SPIRIT

Calm Candies

HERBAL INGREDIENTS

2 teaspoons dried
   passionflower leaf
2 teaspoons dried lemon
   balm leaf
2 teaspoons dried
   chamomile flowers
2 teaspoons dried skullcap
   leaf
rose petal powder (to dust)

Who doesn't love candy? These rose-dusted, 'clean' candies, infused with a synergistic quintet of calming plants, are sweetened only with honey. They are always a hit with the kids. Savour these nectarous, golden-hued jewels, to bring on an instant dose of peacefulness.

METHOD

Make the Candies base recipe (p. 28) with the herbal ingredients.

See Anxiety Protocol (p. 272)

Back to the Land Tea

HERBAL INGREDIENTS

½ teaspoon dried
   Californian poppy aerial
   parts
2 teaspoons dried
   zizyphus fruit/seeds
1 teaspoon dried hops
   flowers
1 teaspoon dried nettle leaf
2 teaspoons dried oat
   straw or milky oat tops

This plant-rich formula aims to guide you back from jarring emotions and experiences. Panic, shock or trauma will often catapult us out of our bodies and cause our nervous systems to go haywire. These sedative nervines really work to bring calm assurance and smooth out hyper-reactive nerves, offering a soft, helping hand. Brew this blend strongly and expect a slightly sleepy, mellow wave to settle in.

METHOD

Make the Medicinal Tea base recipe (p. 33) with the herbal ingredients.

See Trauma/Shock/Panic (p. 292)

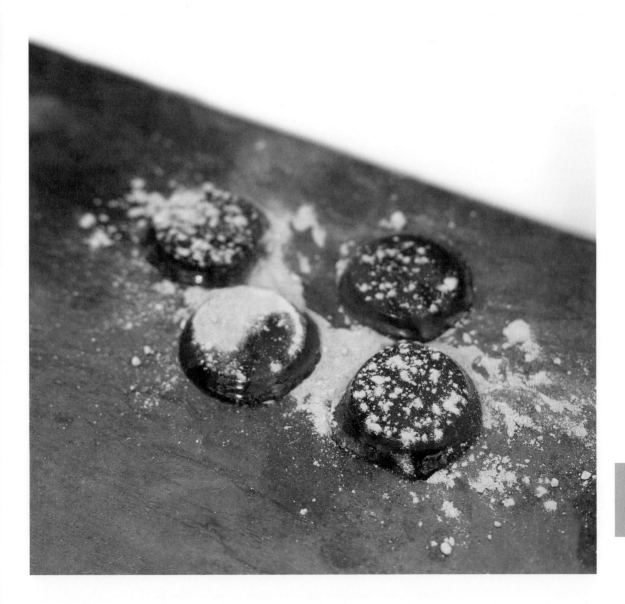

Calm Candies

Chamomile and Lavender Raw Honey

The golden gift of honey mixed with chamomile and lavender offers a sweet, mellow, cloud-like hit to untangle stress, tension and tumultuous emotional/mind states. Spoon into hot water for an instant zen tea, or drizzle over your morning porridge for an extra-soft start to the day.

HERBAL INGREDIENTS

1 tablespoon chamomile
  powder
1 teaspoon lavender
  powder

METHOD

Make the Electuary base recipe (p. 30) with the herbal ingredients.

See Emotional Exhaustion (p. 292)

Calm Nerves Tea

For times when the nervous system feels jittery and overly sensitive, anxiety looms and waves of ungroundedness crash over you. Prepare a strong brew of this soothing tea, sit still with your breath and sip with intention. If experiencing sleeplessness, bring this blend on board as an after-dinner tisane. Nervine-rich herbs are paired with a touch of hibiscus for an easy-to-drink infusion that works to usher in serenity and quell the heaviness within.

HERBAL INGREDIENTS

½ teaspoon dried lavender
2 teaspoons dried lemon
  balm leaf
2 teaspoons dried
  chamomile flowers
2 teaspoons dried skullcap
  leaf
2 teaspoons dried hibiscus
  flowers

METHOD

Make the Medicinal Tea base recipe (p. 33) with the herbal ingredients.

See Anxiety Protocol (p. 272); Depression Protocol (p. 274)

Floral Bath

Sometimes the simplest interventions feel entirely luxurious, and this herbal practice is one of them. Floating in a bath of warm water scattered with precious petals is a treat for the mind, body and spirit. This remedy is perfect for when you may be feeling weary, fatigued, compressed, low and a little lacklustre. When choosing the floral plant portion of the recipe, consider aromatic herbs such as lavender and rose to inspire relaxation and rejuvenation.

HERBAL INGREDIENTS

½–1 cup fresh or dried medicinal flowers (e.g. lavender, calendula, chamomile, rose and rosemary)

METHOD

Mix the flowers and plant material directly into the running bath water – they will float and bob around merrily.

Soak up the serenity for 20 or so minutes.

See Depression Protocol (p. 274)
See also Emotional Exhaustion (p. 292)

Heart of Gold Salve

Imagine a soft, luminous, pink hue trailing over your body as you rub this loving salve over the chest and heart zone. Lush rose- and sunny calendula-infused oils form the basis of this salve, ushering in both a touch of sunny romance and (on the flip side) a supportive golden remedy for heartache, lows and disconnection from self. This salve is simply scented with imbued rose petals and rose geranium and warming cardamom essential oils to support all matters of the heart.

HERBAL INGREDIENTS

½ cup dried rose petals
½ cup dried calendula flowers
45 drops rose geranium essential oil
10 drops cardomom essential oil

METHOD

First, make the Herbal-Infused Oil base recipe (p. 31) with the herbal ingredients.

Now, make the Salve base recipe (p. 36) using your infused oil.

See Depression Protocol (p. 274)
See also Grief (p. 292)

EMOTIONS, MIND, SPIRIT

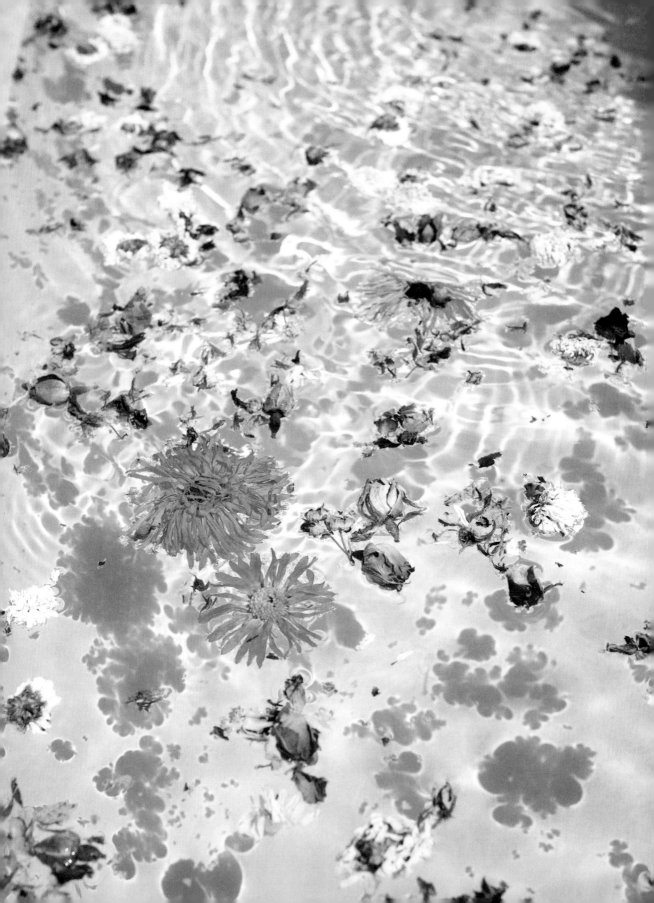

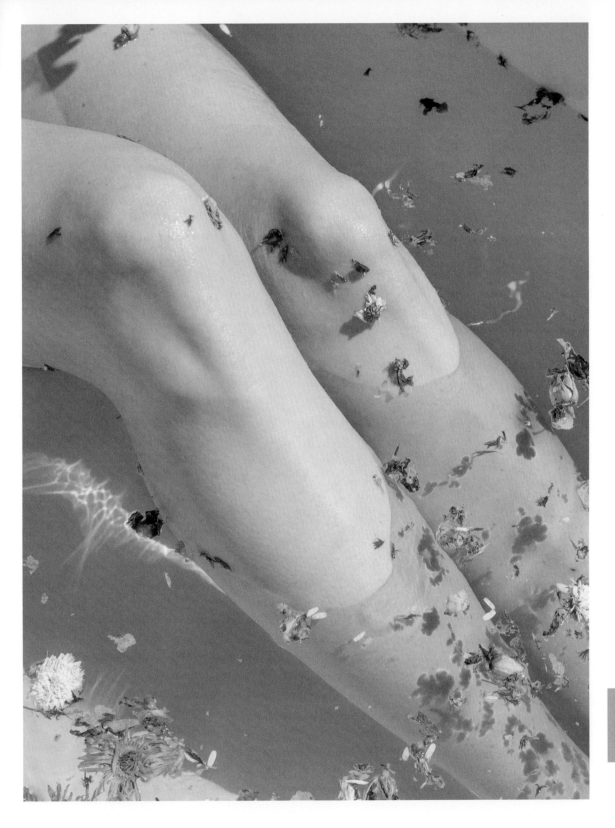

Floral Bath

The Key Tea

HERBAL INGREDIENTS

2 teaspoons dried tulsi
   leaf/flowers
2 teaspoons dried
   hawthorn leaf/berries
1 teaspoon dried rose
   petals/buds
2 ½ teaspoons dried
   cardamom pods

Not just a tea, but a cool oasis that unlocks heated emotional states – an offering of softening for the heart and soul. Rose, hawthorn and cardamom counteract internal anger, frustration and rage while tulsi (otherwise known as the 'incomparable one') lifts the spirit and reshapes the innate stress response, shifting challenging stagnant emotions. This formula is also completely delicious to drink on the daily!

METHOD

Make the Medicinal Tea base recipe (p. 33) with the herbal ingredients.

See Anger (p. 292)

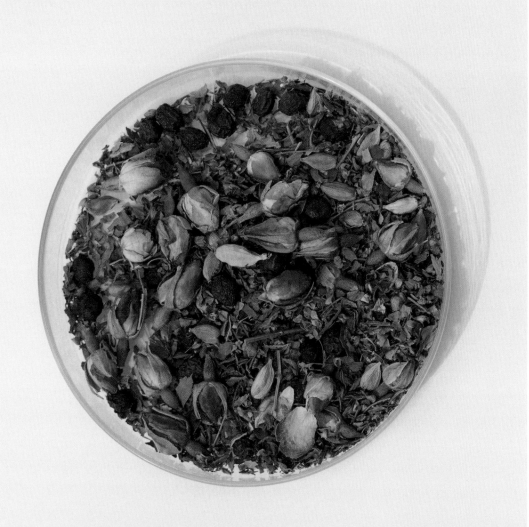

Lion's Mane Tonic

HERBAL INGREDIENTS

1 teaspoon lion's mane
   mushroom powder

1 teaspoon cinnamon
   powder

½ teaspoon cardamom
   powder

½ teaspoon ginger
   rhizome powder

¼ teaspoon maca root
   powder

½ teaspoon lucuma
   powder

a pinch of ground black
   pepper

a dash of raw honey or
   sweetener of choice

For those sluggish mornings or slumpy afternoons where you might find yourself in the thick of fogginess and in need of motivation. This warming blend lights up neurological powers and vitality – in part due to the awesomeness of the medicinal mushroom, lion's mane, which is paired with chai spice tones and adaptogenic maca root. Implement this sustaining treat to renew your capacity for focused endurance.

METHOD

Make the Plant Mylk Tonic base recipe (p. 35) with the herbal ingredients.

See Poor Focus/Cognition Protocol (p. 276)

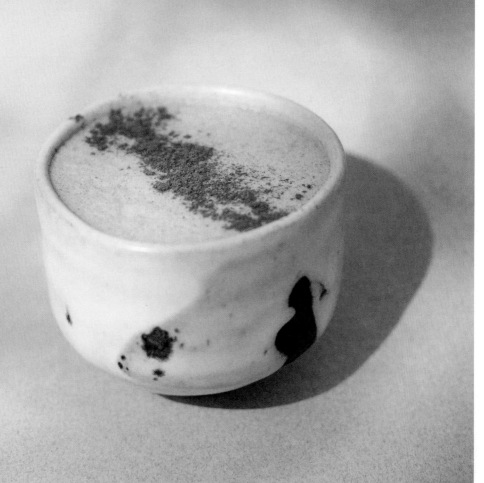

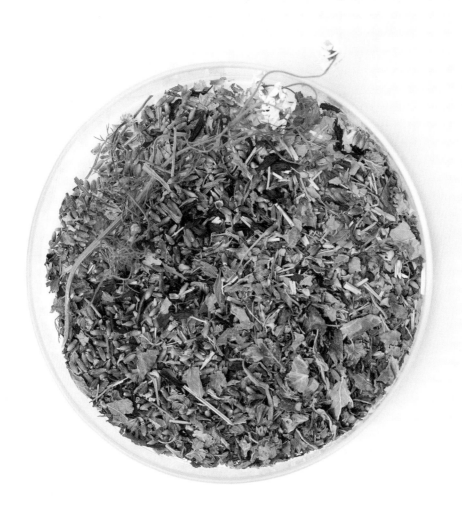

Calm Nerves Tea

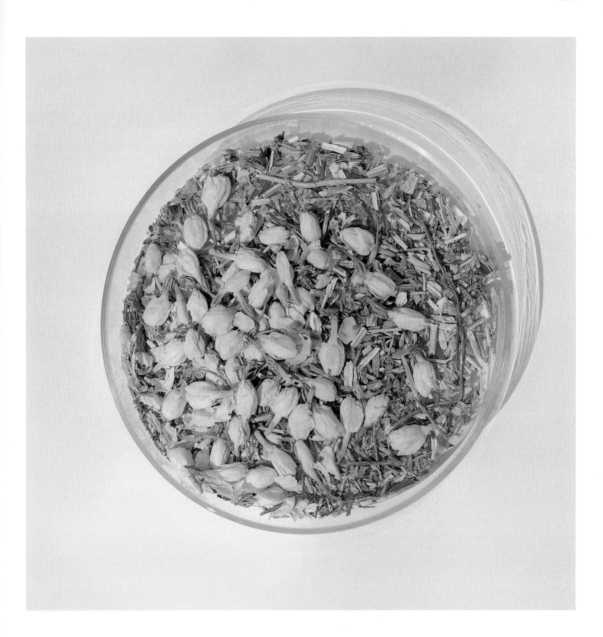

Untangle Tea

Memory Tea

HERBAL INGREDIENTS

2 teaspoons dried brahmi
    leaf
2 teaspoons dried gotu
    kola leaf
2 teaspoons dried ginkgo
    leaf
1 teaspoon dried rosemary
2 teaspoons dried
    peppermint leaf
1 ½ teaspoons dried ginger
    rhizome

Sharpen cognitive function, enhance memory and activate longevity with this blended brain-loving tea. Brahmi and gotu kola, both deeply revered Ayurvedic herbs, create a chalice alongside ginkgo, rosemary, peppermint and ginger to stimulate learning, memory and focus. Truly wonderful to sip on pre-exam, pre-presentation or pre any demanding activity that calls for bolstered brain power.

METHOD

Make the Medicinal Tea base recipe (p. 33) with the herbal ingredients.

See Poor Focus/Cognition Protocol (p. 276)

Peace Within Glycetract

HERBAL INGREDIENTS

¼ cup dried linden flowers
¼ cup dried valerian root
¼ cup dried ashwagandha
    root
½ cup dried passionflower
    leaf
¼ cup dried chamomile
    flowers

A paramount, tranquil, glycerin-based formula to ease marked stress, soothe anxiety and even lull you into the realms of sleep. Consider this blend if restlessness and nervousness are dominant. Adaptogenic ashwagandha pairs beautifully with four prime, herbal, nervous-system remedies, creating a mighty medicinal calming impact.

METHOD

Make the Glycetract Extract base recipe (p. 30) with the herbal ingredients.

DOSAGE

This blend can be dosed throughout the day as needed, and/or dosed a little higher before sleep to support a racing mind and sleeplessness. Follow the suggestions in the dosing guidelines (p. 44).

See Anxiety Protocol (p. 272)
See also Emotional Exhaustion (p. 292)

Tenderness Tea

HERBAL INGREDIENTS

2 teaspoons dried
   rosebuds
2 teaspoons dried
   hawthorn berries
2 teaspoons dried linden
   flowers
2 teaspoons dried
   spearmint leaf

For all matters of the heart, sadness, grief and sorrow. This formula inhabits an empathic energy of compassion and has a settled, soothing kinship with the softest places you can imagine. The perfect blend to offer following a break-up, the loss of a loved one or a heart-to-heart chat. Try a little tenderness.

METHOD

Make the Medicinal Tea base recipe (p. 33) with the herbal ingredients.

See Grief (p. 292)

Untangle Tea

HERBAL INGREDIENTS

2 teaspoons dried anise
   hyssop flowers/leaf
2 teaspoons dried
   motherwort leaf/flowers/
   stem
2 teaspoons dried jasmine
   flowers
2 teaspoons dried vervain
   flowers/leaf

A slightly non-traditional herbal take on a blend for the nervous system, but nevertheless wonderful and effective. In this embodied, gentle blend, motherwort opens her lion-hearted plant powers to pacify stress, soothe anxiety and quieten the body and being – with anise hyssop, vervain and jasmine all playing supporting roles, working towards the same goal. Sip frequently, as needed.

METHOD

Make the Medicinal Tea base recipe (p. 33) with the herbal ingredients.

See Anxiety Protocol (p. 272)

EMOTIONS, MIND, SPIRIT

Rescue Remedies

ANGER

When the heat inside you rises and you quite literally see red, anger permeates within. To unlock and process fiery emotion – with the plants by your side – try **The Key Tea** (p. 284), a heart-centric blend that offers a cooling break.

EMOTIONAL EXHAUSTION

For the frayed and depleted, for the emotionally spent – plant medicines have a profound knack of extending nourishment to those in need, addressing emotional exhaustion holistically. Work with the plants, from adaptogens to nervine-rich herbs, to rebuild resilience. Soak in a bath with **Floral Bath** (p. 281), to calm your body and being. Take a spoonful of **Chamomile and Lavender Raw Honey** (p. 280), or add a spoonful to hot water for an instant calming tea. Or drop a dose of the **Peace Within Glycetract** (p. 290), to nourish and soothe. If you are experiencing sleeplessness, bring the **Slumber Drops** (p. 69) on board.

GRIEF

Being at the mercy of grief feels somewhat like weathering a storm at sea, as relentless tidal waves of emotion wash over you. Grief – she is a dear beast who makes us feel so intensely that it is beyond our powers to suppress our emotions. Feel it, allow it, and keep the plants close by your side. These plant remedies are all heart. Brew a strong pot of **Tenderness Tea** (p. 291), a blend that holds reassurance and softness in all of its floral folds, and sip on it throughout your day or whenever needed. Massage over the chest area with the **Heart of Gold Salve** (p. 281), a rose-embossed balm that brings a sense of serenity and support.

TRAUMA/SHOCK/PANIC

Plant medicines offer a force-field of support for these heightened emotional states. Often when something traumatic is experienced, or re-experienced, the nervous system shifts into reactivity and the cycle of trauma and shock propels us out of our bodies, straight into a state of feeling ungrounded. Try **Back to the Land Tea** (p. 278), a quick-acting, calm, grounding, sedative nervine blend. I find one of the most profound remedies for shock to be Bach's 'Rescue Remedy'. This combination flower essence is available worldwide and is great to have in your first aid kit to use when acute emotions and mind states are present.

Returning to *gratitude*

It is as simple as finding a moment of quietness within. Conjuring up whatever may cause your heart to pulse with gratitude. It may be a place, a person, a colour, a meal, a smell, a feeling.

Hold on to it; this is returning to gratitude.

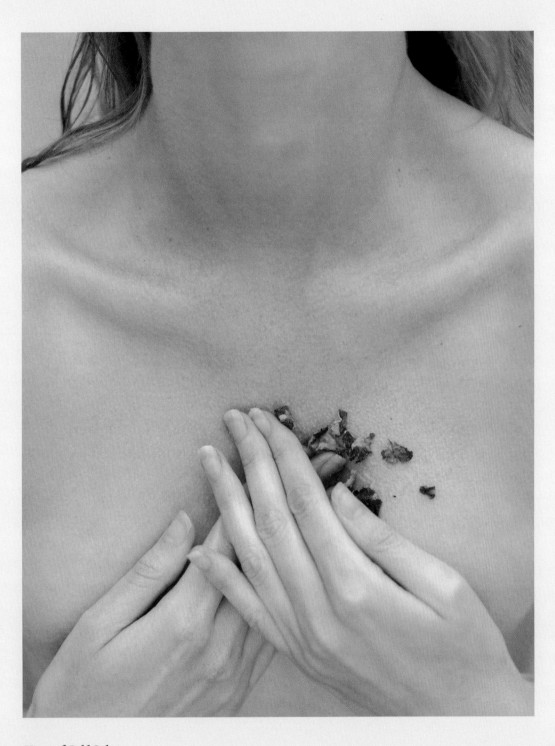

Heart of Gold Salve

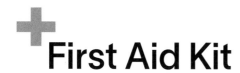
First Aid Kit

BRUISES
_____

Arnica Salve comes to the rescue when you need a speedy way to heal a bruise and relieve tissue trauma.

Arnica Salve

HERBAL INGREDIENTS

⅓ cup dried arnica
   flowers
⅓ cup dried comfrey leaf
⅓ cup dried rosemary

Arnica montana holds a deep affinity for healing bruising and tissue trauma. It is the first plant that herbalists reach for to ameliorate bruising! This overall spectacular salve is a beloved topical recipe to have on hand to aid speedy recovery from bumps, bangs, sprains and wounds – although please be mindful that this salve must not be applied to open wounds. If the wound is open, you could apply the salve to the surrounding area to encourage repair, then smooth it directly onto the affected area once it has healed over. Comfrey and rosemary also lend their relieving properties here.

METHOD

First, make the Herbal-Infused Oil base recipe (p. 31) with the herbal ingredients.

Now, make the Salve base recipe (p. 36) using your infused oil.

BURNS

If you have any fresh aloe vera on hand, break off a juicy leaf and apply the inner gel to a burn asap. Alternatively, the Soothing Salve is perfect, full of St John's wort and lavender, both specifically indicated for burn relief.

Soothing Salve

HERBAL INGREDIENTS

⅓ cup dried St John's wort flowers/leaf
⅓ cup dried calendula flowers
⅓ cup dried lavender

A radically soothing salve for the home herbal first aid kit, perfect for cases of tissue trauma, such as the accidental kitchen cooking burn. Skin-healing plants unite to impart a calming effect when lathered on an acute burn or scrape, encouraging swift healing.

METHOD

First, make the Herbal-Infused Oil base recipe (p. 31) with the herbal ingredients.

Now, make the Salve base recipe (p. 36) using your infused oil.

DOSAGE

Be sure to keep the burn well covered with the salve, reapplying continually.

CUTS/
BLEEDING

Tea tree oil is a potent antiseptic and natural disinfectant, making it perfect for treating cuts. You could use a few drops of pure tea tree oil mixed with coconut oil applied directly to the skin. For minor bleeding, yarrow is the queen of coagulation. Dust the Yarrow Styptic over the area in need and apply pressure. You could also use fresh yarrow leaf, if it is on hand.

Yarrow Styptic

HERBAL INGREDIENT

½–1 cup dried yarrow leaf

Yarrow is an extraordinary blood coagulator, and for this reason alone is an essential plant to grow in any home garden! This plant is a natural pain reliever, offering antimicrobial, anti-inflammatory and wound-healing properties. It is wise to keep a little jar of yarrow powder in your home first aid kit for easy access. For nose bleeds, shaving cuts and everyday accidents that may call for the bandaid approach, consider this yarrow styptic instead to ease blood flow.

METHOD

If picking fresh, allow your yarrow to dry completely before using.

Make the Herbal Powders base recipe (p. 33) with the yarrow leaf. You can store this powder for years to come in a cool, dry, dark cupboard.

Sprinkle ½–1 teaspoon of the yarrow powder onto the area in need. Generally, a little scab will form to seal the bleeding. Leave this be if you can summon up the self control!

EYE STYES

To alleviate and stave off an angry stye, apply a warm Eyebright Wash. It is best to begin this treatment as soon as you feel the stye coming on. Repeat every 2–4 hours from the onset of the stye.

Eyebright Wash

HERBAL INGREDIENTS

2 teaspoons dried chamomile flowers
2 teaspoons dried eyebright leaf/stem/ flowers

An eye stye is essentially a small swollen lump on the edge of the eyelid, which can present as quite sore and angry. Styes are much more common than you may think, and are usually caused by an infection of the tiny oil glands in the eyelid. Catching them early on and applying a warm herbal compress can allow you to shift irritation and inflammation with ease. This herbal practice can be used for all skin concerns involving the sensitive tissues around the eyes.

METHOD

Make the Wash base recipe (p. 39) with the herbal ingredients.

While the wash is still quite warm, saturate a clean washcloth in the warm herbal water. Wring out the excess liquid and apply the warm compress directly onto the closed eye for 5–10 minutes.

DOSAGE

Repeat every 2–4 hours at the onset of stye formation. The frequency of application is critical!

HAEMORRHOIDS

Try the cooling, astringent Cool It Down Salve directly on and around the area of concern. Made with witch hazel, yarrow, gotu kola and butcher's broom, this blend offers relief and healing for the skin.

Cool It Down Salve

HERBAL INGREDIENTS

¼ cup dried witch-hazel
  leaves
¼ cup dried yarrow leaf/
  flowers
¼ cup dried gotu kola leaf
¼ cup dried butcher's
  broom root

Haemorrhoids are the pits – no one would argue with that statement! This herbal blended salve offers support for haemorrhoids and also varicose veins. Apply this salve as needed for internal or external haemorrhoids, and welcome an influx of astringent cooling to ameliorate swollen, red and sore veins.

METHOD

First, make the Herbal-Infused Oil base recipe (p. 31) with the herbal ingredients.

Now, make the Salve base recipe (p. 36) using your infused oil.

HEADACHES

A headache can rear up for many reasons. Sometimes it is simply caused by muscular tension, lack of water or too much screen time. Try these simple interventions to encourage relaxation and release. Rub the Melt Salve onto the site of held tension and surrounding areas – apply liberally. If you have access to a bath, turn the taps on stat, and add the Herbal Magnesium Bath Soak (p. 191), an aromatic delight for the senses made with magnesium-rich Epsom salts. If you do not have access to a bathtub, simply prep a foot bath.

PS: A few helpful prompts. Have you drunk enough water? If not: Hydrate! Hydrate! Hydrate! Check in on whether you have eaten enough grounding food. And how are your stress levels? Do you have any structural muscular tension – can you stretch, roll and massage it away?

Melt Salve

HERBAL INGREDIENTS

⅓ cup dried lavender
⅓ cup dried rosemary
⅓ cup dried St John's
   wort leaf/flowers
25 drops peppermint
   essential oil

Rosemary, lavender and peppermint meet to unlock and disperse held tension, while St John's wort permeates deeply into the skin to relax and unwind muscular discomfort, stress and physical rigidity. This salve is a go-to for headache relief. Simply rub into the temples and across the forehead, and massage deeply into any constricted areas such as the neck and shoulders for sweet relief.

METHOD

First, make the Herbal-Infused Oil base recipe (p. 31) with the herbal ingredients.

Now, make the Salve base recipe (p. 36) using your infused oil.

MUSCULAR
ACHES AND PAINS

For those times when you are feeling structurally achy, stiff and sore, there are plant-rich interventions to tame tension and offer relief. Perhaps you did a heavy workout, or you are experiencing joint pain associated with other symptoms. Rub in the Loosen-Up Liniment, to encourage a reduction in inflammation and support muscular release.

Loosen-Up Liniment

HERBAL INGREDIENTS

2 tablespoons dried chamomile flowers

2 tablespoons dried arnica flowers

2 tablespoons dried peppermint leaf

2 tablespoons dried St John's wort flowers/leaf

2 tablespoons dried rosemary

1 tablespoon dried ginger rhizome

½ teaspoon dried cayenne pepper powder

2 cups witch-hazel extract

10 drops essential oils (optional)

2 tablespoons menthol crystals (optional)

Used aplenty in folk medicine, liniments offer truly fantastic relief for muscular aches and pains, unwinding structural tension and helping to cool internal heat in swollen sore muscles and conditions such as arthritis. They can be formulated with either a cooling action or a heating action, depending on the herbs chosen. Liniments require a highly absorbable base that evaporates with ease when rubbed into the skin, and are traditionally made with rubbing alcohol as the menstruum (or solvent). However, they can also be made with witch-hazel extract, which is what I suggest in the recipe below.

METHOD

Grind all the herbal ingredients into a fine powder and add to a sterilised glass jar. Pour 2 cups of witch-hazel extract over the plant material, ensuring that the herbs are well covered with the liquid.

Seal with an airtight lid and allow it to brew for 4–8 weeks in a warm, sunny spot.

Liniments love a good shake, so every few days give the jar a little shake up.

When the liniment is ready, strain out the plant material through a piece of clean muslin into a sterilised bowl and decant the liquid into a clean spray bottle or sterilised glass jar.

You can add essential oils at this point if desired. Menthol crystals can also be included for an extra cooling impact.

Seal the jar, and label with the date made and ingredients – be sure to always note that this plant medicine is for external use only!

If stored in a cool, dark place, away from sunlight, liniments last for an indefinite period of time.

DOSAGE

Spray or gently rub the liniment into the areas of discomfort, and allow to evaporate. Repeat as needed for muscular relief!

RASHES

Apply the All-Purpose Salve (p. 246) liberally over the rash, to calm irritation and soothe the skin. The quartet of calendula, chickweed, marshmallow root and comfrey aids in reducing inflammation and brings a welcome cooling to any uncomfortable skin woe.

SCRAPES

Pop on the Soothing Salve (p. 295), to aid healing and soothe the skin. Apply liberally, multiple times daily.

SPLINTERS

Soak your embedded splinter in an Epsom salt bath for 15 minutes. Simply fill a basin with warm water and a heaped tablespoon of Epsom salts. The salts create osmotic pressure on the skin, the idea being that the water in your body will diffuse across the membrane of your skin, out towards the concentrated solution of Epsom salts. This helps to draw out the splinter, making it much easier to remove.

SPRAINS

Apply Arnica Salve (p. 294) throughout the day, to ease trauma and support soft-tissue recovery.

STINGS AND BITES

A herbalist's quick trick in the garden is to reach for a ribwort (*Plantago lanceolata*) leaf, chew it up a little and apply it directly to the affected area. A lo-fi poultice of sorts, this quickly neutralises any itching or stinging sensation. You could also use the All-Purpose Salve (p. 246) or the Soothing Salve (p. 295) to calm any irritation.

SUNBURN

For quick, cooling relief, spray on the Sunburn Mist – a strong infusion of spearmint tea and green tea. For longer-term healing, seal moisture into the skin with either fresh aloe vera or the Soothing Salve (p. 295).

Sunburn Mist

HERBAL INGREDIENTS

2 tablespoons dried
    spearmint leaf
2 tablespoons dried green
    tea leaf

It can be frighteningly easy to lull the day away in the sunshine, only to discover once you're back inside that you have a gnarly case of sunburn. Essentially this mix is a cooled tea, entirely easy to prepare, which is simply spritzed liberally all over your body to calm the sun's effects. Green tea and spearmint both hold an affinity for mitigating the impacts of sunburn, and bring a menthol-fresh wave of relief.

METHOD

Make the Medicinal Tea base recipe (p. 33) with the herbal ingredients and allow the tea to cool in the fridge.

Once cool, decant the tea into a spray bottle, shake well to combine and spray all over the skin onto areas in need. Repeat frequently!

TOOTHACHE

Apply Clove Oil (p. 97) to the affected gum and tooth for natural numbing relief. To manage associated pain, dose the analgesic Sweet Relief Tincture as needed.

Sweet Relief Tincture

HERBAL INGREDIENTS

2 tablespoons dried Californian poppy aerial parts
¼ cup dried mugwort leaf
½ cup dried passionflower leaf
¼ cup dried valerian root
2 tablespoons dried corydalis root

When pain is rife, this is the tincture to reach for. A gentle heads-up – this is a STRONG concoction! Laden with analgesic, anodyne and nervine sedative herbals, it is ideal for nerve pain such as dental or back pain, and extreme emotional unease such as anxiety, panic attacks and hysteria. This blend works to numb and downgrade pain in all of its uncomfortable manifestations.

METHOD

Make the Tincture base recipe (p. 38) with the herbal ingredients.

DOSAGE

Use only as needed. Start with a lower drop dosage to check for sensitivity, and work up from there as outlined in the dosing guidelines (p. 45).

UTI (URINIARY TRACT INFECTION)

Cranberry juice and water are known allies in combating urinary tract infections, but so are many other incredible plant medicines. It is best to implement this protocol immediately upon sensing the onset of UTI symptoms. Prep a pot of Corn Silk Tea, an incredibly simple brew made with the silky threads of the corn ear; this is a soothing diuretic, indicated for urinary tract infections. Dose the Acute UTI Tincture, and once acute symptoms ease, drink 2–3 cups of Kidney Tone Tea daily, for follow-up kidney and bladder support – and to replenish and nurture.

PS: Pump up probiotic-rich foods (see p. 20) to support healthy urogenital-tract flora. Increasing your intake of fermented foods, such as cultured yoghurts and kefir, will aid gut health, which is interconnected with urinary tract health. If you are getting frequent UTIs, it is super important to work on improving your overall gut health.

Acute UTI Tincture

HERBAL INGREDIENTS

½ cup dried echinacea root/leaf/seeds/flowers
¼ cup dried uva ursi leaf
¼ cup dried olive leaf
¼ cup dried marshmallow root
¼ cup dried chamomile flowers

To combat any looming urinary tract infection, take this blend at the onset of even the slightest niggle of urinary tract discomfort. If you tend towards getting UTIs, this is a great tincture to have in your home apothecary. Demulcent marshmallow root meets immune-enhancing echinacea and olive leaf, while in the background uva ursi works to downgrade and eradicate microbial build-up in the urinary tract.

METHOD

Make the Tincture base recipe (p. 38) with the herbal ingredients.

DOSAGE

UTI symptoms are generally very acute, so dose accordingly, as outlined in the dosing guidelines (p. 45).

Corn Silk Tea

HERBAL INGREDIENT

silk from 1–2 fresh corn
    husks

Kitchen herbalism at its finest! Humble corn offers a wealth of healing for the bladder and urinary tract. The fine, silky strands of the inner husk are simply peeled away and boiled to release an extraordinarily soothing potion, which can be used to treat UTIs, as well as associated concerns such as kidney stones, prostate issues and enuresis (incontinence). The benefits of this tea extend to support for the cardiovascular system and normalisation of cholesterol levels, as well as the treatment of high blood pressure and diabetes!

METHOD

Make the Decoction base recipe (p. 29) with the corn silk.

Kidney Tone Tea

HERBAL INGREDIENTS

1 teaspoon dried burdock
    root
1 teaspoon dried buchu
    leaf
1 teaspoon dried cleavers
    leaf/seeds/stem
1 teaspoon dried horsetail
    aerial parts

A primo blend for the kidneys, bringing tonification, replenishment and purification. Employ this soothing and anti-inflammatory tea to support urinary/bladder infections and irritations, or bring it on post-infection for continued care and revitalisation. There is a gentle diuretic and cleansing action woven within this formula, which works to clear kidney stagnancy and enhance detoxification of these key waste-removal organs.

METHOD

Make the Medicinal Tea base recipe (p. 33) with the herbal ingredients.

Index

Remedy Recipes and Protocols are indicated in bold.

Acknowledgements

Noah, this book begins and ends with you. As I wrote, tested recipes and agonised over the details, you designed by my side, breathing life into every page. Thank you for graciously supporting me and encouraging me to walk this plant path, and for holding every incarnation, vision and creation I set my sights on. Thank you for making the space to allow this book to hold us captive for over a year! Your patience, virgo mastery and good nature baffle me in the best possible way. Thank you for being my person in love and creation. Thank you for loving me so mightily.

To Kirsten Abbott – taking this second book trip with you as my publisher has been a true delight. Thank you for your eternal support, sound advice and warmth. Your commitment to the work is nothing short of impressive, and your genuine care for me and my message means the actual world. All that I have produced in print is thanks to you; thank you for finding me.

To Sam Palfreyman, thank you for your focused energy, wonderful work and openness to dive into an ambitious project and learn the language of the plants. You are now an honorary herbalist in my eyes!

Thank you to the wonderful team at Thames & Hudson. What a team you are. I'm proud to call Thames & Hudson my home.

To Georgia Blackie: collaborating with you again to create another book has been a dream. You possess an incredible ability to nimbly adapt to whatever part of nature you capture, be it a person or a plant. Thank you for all of the visual beauty that you've brought to my books, for being my dear friend who is always open to listening, and for forever conjuring up tangible plans to move forward that are always simply perfect.

Some of the vessels and wares photographed in the book were lent or created by my absolute favourite people. Thank you to Jasmine Christie of Anamundi Studio for always lending me boxes overflowing with props, and to my dear Chanel Tobler and Maya Bartlett, for allowing me to grace these pages with your work – they are some of my most beloved ceramics.

To my darling friend Ema Taylor Rabbidge, for lending me your time, energy and contagious spirit as well as your beautiful being, which was captured in many of the images. To Maddy and Jimmy, thank you for welcoming us into your forest and into that outrageously ideal outdoor bathtub. Thank you doubly, Maddy, for being willing to jump into said bathtub and be scattered with flowers – you are a true gem. To our sweet Sage, thank you for your gentle little hands. And to Jume, thank you for opening up your magical homestead on the creek, I am so happy we could share a few treasured shots from your beautiful wooden oasis.

Many warm, wholehearted thanks must go to Sarah Mann, Justina Edwards, Lauren Haynes and Jacqui Bushell for picking up my calls always, for hearing my herbal thoughts and process, for sharing your plant wisdoms and for easing any concerns I may be holding. My trusted herbal community, I thank you endlessly.

To my sweet herbal helpers: you all showed up with such enthusiasm and love of the plants, making it a delight to test hundreds of recipes with you all. Thank you, dear Ruby, Taylor, Katie, Amanda, Annabel, Ebany, Holly, Morgan, Bronte and Helena.

So many friends held me and cheered me on in the process of creating this book. Thank you all for your enduring encouragement and love. Extreme love goes out to you Lula, thank you for always being my BFF, which I will keep referring to you as even when we are 95 years wise. When I was super stretched in the process of writing, you listened and loved me. Indigo Sparke, thank you for speaking my language. Ashley Neese, thank you for the deep kinship as we walk these wild parallel paths. Katie Dalebout, the space you hold in the space between the space is everything. Love you so. To Dominic Kuneman, my other favourite earth sign, thank you for your fine eye and friendship. And a very special extension of gratitude must also go out to you Jordanna Levin, for always being my friend first and foremost, as well as a fellow author full of seriously good advice.

Mum and dad, thanks for supporting me in my pursuit of this green path of mine and trusting that I would one day find my deep purpose, no matter how unconventional it might be – which I know you both completely anticipated! Your love and support has truly shaped how I walk in the world. To my brother, Luke, thank you for the heart-to-hearts, they always fill me with belonging.

I must also share my sincere gratitude for the ever-cosy old, converted church house I currently call home on Bundjalung country. I have now written two books cocooned in your sweet old bones. And to you Clark and Quinn, for keeping me company and reminding me to play, throw you balls and take you for walks. You always seem to know when a break is much needed.

Warm thanks to my clients, who have entrusted me with their precious healing journeys and in turn shaped the very fabric of who I am as a practitioner and person, deeply influencing my ability to create this book.

And finally, to you, dear readers. Thank you for the love and support you gave my first book, the way you so warmly received it means the world to me. Thank you for finding your way to this very place, with this book in hand. May this creation be just what you need, may the power of the plants help you recalibrate to your own beautiful beat and may they remind you that you too are an integral part of the symphony of nature.

Bestselling author of *Plants for the People*, Erin Lovell Verinder is the voice of contemporary plant medicine. She runs a bustling digital clinic helping clients back to health. Erin lives, works and gardens in the wilds of the Byron Bay hinterland.

The Plant Clinic is her second book.

Join Erin on the plant path at @erinlovellverinder.

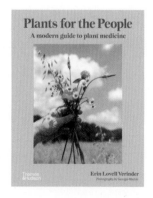

First published in Australia in 2021
by Thames & Hudson Australia Pty Ltd
11 Central Boulevard, Portside Business Park
Port Melbourne, Victoria 3207
ABN: 72 004 751 964

First published in the United States of America in 2021
by Thames & Hudson Inc.
500 Fifth Avenue
New York, New York 10110

First published in the United Kingdom in 2022
by Thames & Hudson Ltd
181a High Holborn
London WC1V 7QX

The Plant Clinic © Thames & Hudson Australia 2021

Text © Erin Lovell Verinder
Images © Georgia Blackie

24 23 22 21   5 4 3 2 1

Thames & Hudson Australia wishes to acknowledge that
Aboriginal and Torres Strait Islander people are the first
storytellers of this nation and the traditional custodians of
the land on which we live and work. We acknowledge their
continuing culture and pay respect to Elders past, present
and future.

ISBN 978-1-760-76141-7 (hardback)
ISBN 978-1-760-76172-1 (U.S. edition)

A catalogue record for this
book is available from the
National Library of Australia

British Library Cataloguing-in-Publication Data
A catalogue record for this book is available from the
British Library

Library of Congress Control Number 2021935532

Every effort has been made to trace accurate ownership
of copyrighted text and visual materials used in this book.
Errors or omissions will be corrected in subsequent editions,
provided notification is sent to the publisher.

On the front: Spring Elixir, *see p. 143*
On the back: Collecting calendula

Design: Noah Harper Checkle
Editing: Diana Hill

Printed and bound in China by 1010 Printing International
Limited.

Be the first to know about our new releases,
exclusive content and author events by visiting
thamesandhudson.com.au
thamesandhudson.com
thamesandhudsonusa.com

FSC® is dedicated to the promotion of responsible forest
management worldwide. This book is made of material from
FSC®-certified forests and other controlled sources.

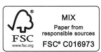

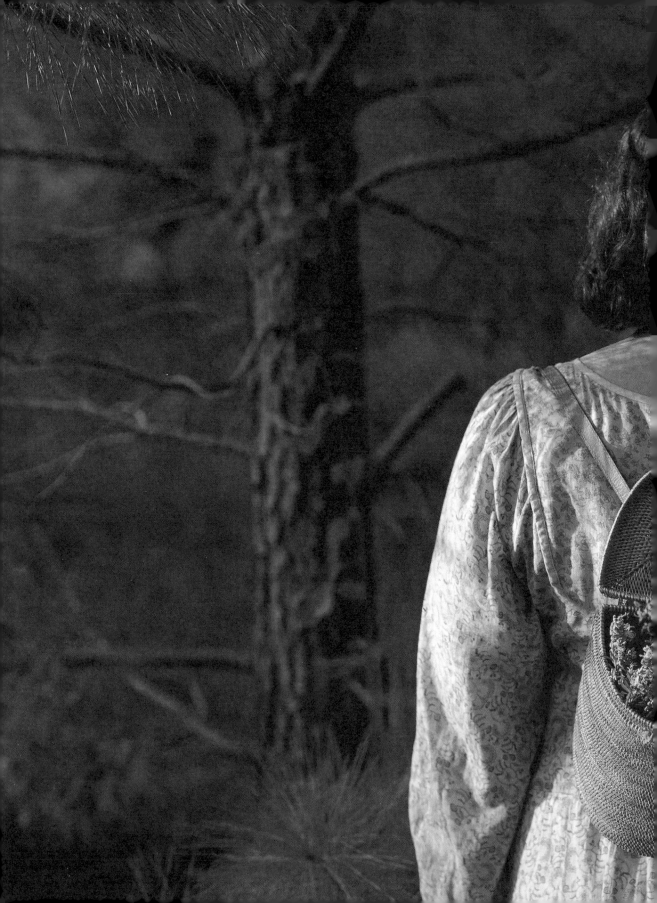